I0520619

THE 12-STEP GUIDE FOR SKEPTICS

Clearing Up Common Misconceptions of a Path to Sobriety

A R L I N A   A

Copyright In Progress 2024 by Arlina A.

Library of Congress Cataloging in Publication Data

ISBN: 979-8-9913088-0-9 (paperback)

Website: https://www.the12stepguideforskeptics.com

DEDICATION

For my family:
Bobby, Travis and Tyler. I love you best in the world.

Scott & Maureen for your constant unconditional love.

In loving memory of
Aida Messersmith
Frank L. Messersmith

CONTENTS

PART 3: Overcoming Common Barriers to Entry – Myths, Misperceptions, and Truths About 12-Step Programs

PART 4: Reasons People Leave

PART 5: Taking Action

START HERE

WHY DO YOU NEED THIS GUIDE ANYWAY?

Well, that is for you to decide! But in this guide, you will gain context and perspectives to help you challenge common obstacles people face when thinking about joining a 12-Step program—or even staying in one. The goal is to help you complete the steps; gain control over alcohol; and practice a plan for living a thriving, peaceful life, without alcohol.

This Guide is For You If:

- You are thinking about using a 12-Step program to quit drinking.
- You are looking for support and community on your alcohol-free journey.
- You've tried a 12-Step program and left, but you're thinking about giving it another try.
- You know someone who is struggling with drinking, and you want to encourage them to try the 12-Step process.

Before we get started, I want to state the three guiding tenets of this guide

1. The 12 steps are a worthy endeavor that can lead to a profound transformation and a whole new way of life.
2. This guide is meant to provide you with context and perspectives to challenging ideas so you can make progress and complete the steps in order with the help of a sponsor.
3. **The people are not the program.** I cannot overstate this point enough! The steps (aka the program) and the peo-

ple at meetings <u>are two distinctly separate components</u>. They are intended to work together, but keep in mind that people in general are flawed, and no one person represents the official organization. It's important to find people that you can relate to and that can take time. Be persistent and patient.

What you will NOT find in these pages:

- Claims that the 12-Step program is the only way to achieve sobriety and long-term happiness.
- Promises that if you complete the 12 steps you will stay sober forever.
- Warnings that if you stop going to meetings you will certainly relapse.

PART 1

The Overview

The Fine Print

If you are physically addicted to alcohol and/or drugs, please seek medical attention. This book is for educational purposes only.

The steps from the first edition (1939) of Alcoholics Anonymous, which is now in public domain. The opinions in this book are mine alone. I do not represent Alcoholics Anonymous or any other 12-Step program. This book is not a replacement for going to meetings or working the steps with a sponsor. My opinions are heavily biased toward the 12-Step program as it has helped me stay sober since 4/23/94. The process of attending meetings, reading the literature, working the steps with a sponsor, and helping others to achieve sobriety, has profoundly and positively altered the trajectory of my life.

2

Welcome to the Journey

The journey to sobriety and the path beyond can be challenging at times, but full of incredible surprises. If you choose this path, then buckle up! It's going to be a bumpy ride, but totally worth it.

My intention with this book is to offer my experiences and perspectives and add context to the culture presented within the 12-Step program. I also hope to debunk many common myths and misperceptions about the program. No program is perfect, so while I will validate some of the challenging aspects of it, I can also offer a safe path forward.

My hope is to remove the barriers preventing you from going through the process and thereby receiving life-changing benefits.

If at the end of this book, you decide 12-Step programs are not for you, that's okay too. There are many paths to recovery, and a vast pool of resources from which to draw.

The point is to break free from alcohol so that you can start living up to your fullest potential.

For simplicity's sake, I will be focusing on alcoholism—aka. alcohol-use disorder—and will refer to addiction in general terms.

If you've fallen into addiction, try not to be too hard on yourself. You can't hate yourself well. I believe the purpose of any addiction is to distract us from emotional pain. What starts out as a coping mechanism can easily cross over into addiction. It's the underlying emotional pain that is the root cause of addiction and that is what needs to be healed.

One of the many benefits of the 12-Step program is that it effectively kick-starts the healing journey. Breaking free of alcohol is just the beginning. It can help you to process emotional pain to resolution so that it does not continue to drive unhealthy behaviors—and provides you with tools and support to create a life you love.

We now know addiction is not a moral issue, and it should be treated with empathy and compassion. Do those in the grip of addiction do things that are immoral? Absolutely. However, those struggling with addiction are typically more focused on avoiding their own pain rather than intentionally causing it in others. The 12 steps are very effective at resolving the associated guilt and shame that result from addiction.

Addiction is a complex, multi-faceted issue with many variables; it can be thought of as a spectrum ranging from mild to extreme obsession. Everyone is different, which is why there are so many modalities for treating and healing addiction in all its forms. Unfortunately, many of these treatments are costly and inaccessible to those who need them the most. The good news is that 12-Step programs are widely available at little to no cost and—with hard work and persistence—are incredibly effective in facilitating change.

3

A Fresh Perspective

If you came to me and asked, "I think I need to quit drinking. What would you recommend?" Without hesitation I would say, "Go to an AA meeting and work the 12 steps with a sponsor." But that wouldn't be all. I would suggest we meet for coffee so I could give you some pointers and clarify a few things, especially if you're feeling skeptical or apprehensive.

I mean, who wouldn't be skeptical these days? Although AA is supposed to be an anonymous program, there's a lot that has been said about it on social media and in TV shows, movies, books, and magazine articles. A lot of it is not so flattering. It's no wonder you might be skeptical. Especially if you read the steps and take it at face value without the supporting context as I did.

When I got sober in 1994, I had little exposure to AA—or "the program" as it's commonly referred to. My mom had dated a sober guy named Al when I was 14. He was a nice guy who went to AA; he took us to an AA picnic which was an eye-opening experience to say the least. They held a meeting and a speaker walked up onto the stage.

He was an older gentleman who had been sober for decades. His name was Jack and he told a story about how he would drink with his bird, Petey, who had his own shot glass of whiskey. Jack told everyone how the bird would get drunk and chase the dog around the house and everyone laughed. He was also one of the most inspiring and eloquent speakers I had ever heard. Jack was so vulnerable and transparent as he talked about how bad his drinking had been. He shared how hopeless he had felt toward the end, but that someone from AA shared their story of recovery and it gave him hope that he could quit drinking too. Jack joined AA and was so profoundly changed by the experience of working the steps with a sponsor, that he dedicated his life to carrying AA's message of hope to others.

When Jack was done speaking, the meeting facilitator stepped up to the microphone and asked if anyone was celebrating a milestone. A young woman, not much older than I was, came forward. She said her name was Tammy, she was an alcoholic, was 90 days sober and took a chip from the facilitator. I was shocked. I didn't know girls her age could suffer from alcoholism.

Afterwards I didn't think about it much. I was only 14 and had just started to drink. I didn't think what they were saying applied to me because I didn't think I had a problem.

That was the extent of my direct exposure to AA. Years later when I found myself struggling with alcohol, it didn't even occur to me to go to a meeting. Honestly, I didn't think alcohol was really the problem. I thought my problems were because of my family, romantic relationships, friends, work stress, and a lack of money.

To be fair, there wasn't anything remotely relatable in mainstream media like there is today. In 1992 when I started to question my drinking, there were no memoirs from women like me talking about how they quit drinking by going to AA—or any other method for that matter. Now there are so many there's even a name for that genre. The cool kids call it "Quit Lit" which is short for 'quit literature.'

So in 1994—when I was finally ready to get sober—I asked my colleague and friend, Mitch, for help. I knew he was sober because I had been telling him about my drinking escapades. He would patiently listen to me and share how he used to drink like I did, but quit by going to AA. When I finally asked him what he thought I should do about my drinking, he suggested we go to a meeting together so I could see what it was like for myself.

I didn't really want to but by then I felt utterly defeated and was tired of trying to quit on my own. I told Mitch I was nervous about who might see me and the kind of people that would be there. He told me not to worry; that there would be people like us there. He suggested I introduce myself as an alcoholic when they asked for newcomers. He said I didn't have to talk if I didn't want to, but I should get phone numbers from some of the women. He said the women would be the ones to help me moving forward because it was recommended that women work with women.

I am very grateful to Mitch for inviting me and sitting with me at that first meeting. I don't know if I would have gone by myself. To be honest, even though I had a friend with me, showing up was still very uncomfortable. I felt stiff and awkward, like a deer caught in the headlights.

Looking back, it would have been nice to have a guidebook to help me navigate some of the customs, how to interact with the members, or even what was expected of me as a newly sober person. I didn't retain much of what they said from that first meeting, but I do remember the feelings. I felt welcomed, safe, and hopeful. Like maybe there was something to this thing after all. That maybe it isn't what I thought it was.

People who are getting sober today are not doing it in the same world I got sober in. There is a lot of exposure to AA through mainstream media, and even more so on social media. Due to the tradition of members being anonymous, it seems like a lot of the people who talk about AA are the ones who have negative things to say about it.

When I hear specific criticisms, they are typically based on bad experiences with a few of the members who—in all fairness—are not always healthy but they do not represent the entire community or the program itself. I have also heard criticisms founded on misunderstandings of the literature; for example, the idea that we are powerless, when in fact it is saying we are powerless <u>over alcohol</u>. Or when people see the word 'God' and assume it's a religious program, when in fact it is based on spiritual principles.

I usually think, *Wow, with some boundaries, some additional context, and a shift in perspective they could move past these common barriers and gain access to all the amazing benefits of the program.*

All the negative exposure to AA has fueled widespread misconceptions, potentially deterring people who could benefit greatly from working through the steps.

This is my attempt at not only clearing up some common misunderstandings, but also to provide the guidance I wish I had when I first got sober.

Listen, getting sober is scary. Personally I was terrified to give up the one thing that always brought me relief. I was actively looking for reasons *not* to go to AA. Eventually, after trying everything else I could think of and not being able to quit, the pain of not going became greater than the fear of giving it a try.

Before we went to the meeting, Mitch shared the acronym H.O.W. which stands for Honesty, Open-Mindedness, and Willingness. He suggested that if I could adopt a HOW mindset, I could attend meetings, follow the suggestions, work through the steps with a sponsor, and learn to stay sober. That's the advice I want to pass along to you too.

I would also suggest that you study the literature yourself to understand the suggestions and culture which are often misinterpreted, even by members. There are two main books, *Alcoholics Anonymous* (also known as the "Big Book") and *The Twelve Steps and Twelve Traditions*, but there are also a lot of pamphlets that cover things like the use of medication, sponsorship, how to run a meeting, and other important topics. Remember that members can have strong opinions that may or may not reflect the official position of the organization, so it's important to know the difference.

The fact is that the 12 steps saved my life. My drinking had escalated to the point where I was binge drinking on a regular basis, blacking out, driving drunk, and putting myself and others in danger. Not to mention the damage I was inflicting on my self-esteem.

For example, one morning I woke up after a particularly bad night of heavy drinking and went out front to see if my truck was in the driveway. I had completely blacked out and figured there was a 50% chance of it being there. It was, but what I found were huge weeds sticking out of the space between the front of the hood and the fender. I had a vague recollection of overshooting the freeway offramp and driving into the weeds, but no memory of how I got home. The shock of how reckless I had been sent a chill down my spine. It was a miracle I didn't kill myself in a car accident or hurt anyone else. But that didn't stop me from drinking again. I just told myself I wouldn't drink so much the next time.

And it wasn't just the drunk driving. When I went out drinking with my friends, there was no way of predicting my behavior or which alter ego would come out to play. I dubbed them Wimpy Wendy and Badass Betsy because when I got really drunk, I was either crying or fighting. Sometimes both. Actually, years later I realized there was a third alter ego: Slutty Susan. Everyone LOVED her…literally.

In any case, I would wake up the next morning so humiliated by the way I behaved. I was unrecognizable even to myself. And that was just the parts I could remember. Most of the time I would hear about what I had done from my friends the next day. Their reactions were mixed. They would either be really pissed at me for ruining their night or just flat-out disgusted. In the end, I had no friends left. They didn't want to hang out with me anymore and I couldn't blame them. There came a point when I was always on the hunt for new friends who didn't know how unpredictable or out of control I was when I drank. I hated who I had become. It was such a lonely and isolating period of my life. I felt utterly lost and broken.

Toward the end, I would drink so much that I would get sick and vomit almost every time I drank. I used to make light of that by saying if I didn't have splash marks on my shoes, it wasn't a good time. Classy, I know.

It was unpredictable as to when it would happen too. Once I got alcohol poisoning at a San Francisco Giants baseball game. I was with a bunch of fancy corporate guys I met at the restaurant I worked at. They had invited me to ride with them on a private party bus with their coworkers. On the way to the ballpark, I drank so much I threw up at the table inside the bar in front of everyone. The guys I was with all abandoned me and somehow, I ended up in a first aid room inside the stadium. Since I didn't know where they were sitting, the first aid people took me to the parking lot to find the bus I rode up in. I had to sit in front of the bus because they wouldn't let me inside for fear I'd get sick in there too. That's when Wimpy Wendy showed up. I cried throughout that whole experience. I cried the whole way home on the bus because I was so drunk and embarrassed. Not so surprising, those guys never came back to the restaurant. It was such a deeply humiliating experience that the thought of it keeps me from drinking to this day.

On those long and painful nights when I was sick, I would press my face on the cold tile floor in my bathroom, feeling too nauseous to move too far from the toilet. My head spinning and my throat burning from all the vomiting. By late afternoon when I was finally able to drag myself out of bed and look in the mirror, I looked like hell. I'd have these little red dots under my eyes. I found out that there's a name for that. Petechiae. It means there was so much pressure in my face from vomiting that the blood vessels under my eyes ruptured.

Listen, that's just the tip of the insanity iceberg. I had many nights like that, but I'm not going to pretend I didn't have any fun. I had A LOT of fun. I have so many wild stories of things my friends and I did when we were drunk. Some that still make me giggle; but looking back—after you reach a certain age—it's just not cute anymore. The truth is that at the end of my drinking days, life felt so dark and hopeless I began to consider ways to end it all.

Obviously, that didn't happen. Because of a few caring people, I found sobriety instead.

The scary thing is, I almost missed out on my sobriety because the program isn't what I thought it was going to be: a sad, shameful group of dingy church basement dwellers. I mean sometimes it's that, but to my surprise even those meetings have moments of profound insight and wisdom that made me feel hopeful. At most of the meetings I attended, I found people struggling with the same feelings of confusion, frustration, or inadequacy I was. With the same desires for a better life doing their best to be better people. I met people from all walks of life in those meetings: everyone from those fresh out of prison or rehab, to high-powered corporate executives, authors, doctors, nurses, nuns, and lawyers. I met brilliant artists, teachers, construction workers, singers, and movie producers. People with a wicked sense of humor and a gift for storytelling. People who were generous, selfless, and kind. I have had amazing experiences and developed unique and priceless friendships over the three decades that I have attended meetings.

Using the principles of the program, I created the life of my dreams. I have had an amazing career in high-tech sales in Silicon Valley, married the love of my life, and we raised two wonderful young men who have never seen me drunk. I have a wealth of friends and my life has purpose and meaning. I am in a unique position to be of service to those trying to quit drinking, because I know how it feels to be unable to control it.

There's so much I want to share with anyone considering undertaking the 12 steps that I feel compelled to put it into this guidebook.

The overarching goal of this guide is to help you find a way to complete all the steps with the help of a sponsor and stay sober.

When you first read the steps, it might not be obvious how they will help you quit drinking. It wasn't obvious to me. The first time I read them, I thought, *Okay now what?* I had real problems and I didn't get how the steps were going to solve them. If it hadn't been for Mitch, it would have been easy for me to dismiss them. He told me reading them isn't the same as working them with a sponsor and that through the process, I would be able to address all my issues.

In all fairness, I can see why some people are quick to dismiss the program. Some of the language is triggering and some of the ideas are outdated. The field of recovery has advanced a tremendous amount since AA was founded. I understand why you might have already concluded that it won't work for you, but I'm going to ask you to hold off on deciding against it until you have more information. There is value in getting curious and learning more about the whole program before you decide.

There is a parable from *The Power of Now* by Eckhart Tolle that illustrates the point of how curiosity can lead you to unexpected and surprising realizations. In the parable, a man walks past a beggar on the street who is sitting on an old box. The beggar asks the man for some change, but the man says he has nothing to give. Then the man asks, "What's inside that box you're sitting on?" The beggar says, "Nothing, it's just an old box I've been sitting on for years." The man encourages the beggar to look inside and to his amazement, the box was full of treasure all along.

From a lot of people's perspective, the moral of the story is that most of us look outside ourselves for what we need, and that the real treasure lies in unexpected places. While on the surface I agree, I also see another lesson in this parable. In the narrative, there is an obstacle between the beggar and what he desired—the beggar's own interpretation of the box. He saw the box only as a worthless object, merely a stool, something to rest upon.

Yet in his haste to categorize it, he missed its true value. Without curiosity or investigation, the beggar came to an incomplete conclusion. Not only that but he viewed the object with contempt. He had what is known in the AA literature as contempt prior to investigation. He was relying on his own uninformed conclusion without even realizing it and he nearly missed out on the treasure. Without curiosity, it is all too easy to relegate something (or someone) to a place of little importance.

As the parable goes, he did eventually find the treasure—but how much time was wasted in needless suffering? Would his life, relationships, and experiences have been more peaceful, loving, and fulfilling had he simply been more curious?

Sometimes words are like that box. At face value, they appear as something we think we understand. In truth and in practice, words are symbols we assign meaning to but we rarely stop to consider whether our definitions are complete—or even our own.

When people look at the 12 steps and see words like "God," "powerless," and "alcoholic," it's easy to assume they know what that means. I know I did. But through the lens of recovery, these words have additional context which creates new meaning. The context is the critical piece that makes all the difference in making an informed decision.

This is why it's important to speak with others who have been through the process themselves and can provide context. Their definition of God might be vastly different than yours. They might tell you how their understanding of powerlessness over alcohol freed them of it. They no longer waste time and energy trying to manage it. You might also reconsider the meaning of the word "alcoholic," and how to some it is a badge of honor. To those who know what it's like to muster the courage to go from hopelessness to empowerment, it's as far as you can get from a so-called shame label.

I want to acknowledge an important paradox here. While I suggest you talk to people with experience, I also want to caution you against total reliance on other members. It's important to seek answers to specific challenges from people who have already overcome them, but they won't always have the right answer for you. In time, you will know when you have the right answer, because when you get quiet it will resonate in your heart and in your gut. Trust that feeling. It is your guiding compass.

I have a confession to make. I was like the beggar in the parable when I first started my 12-Step journey. I saw the word "God" and nearly rejected the program right then and there. The God I knew wasn't going to help me. After all, I had been asking that God to fix me my whole life, yet I constantly felt like a failure. Ultimately, I just gave up on it. It didn't work for me.

Even though I was desperate to stop drinking, and in my darkest hour I whispered into the void for this "God" to help me one more time. When those feelings of desperation subsided, I knew I couldn't go back to the religious God of my childhood. That God was judgmental, punishing, and downright confusing. On one hand I was taught that God's love was so great my puny human mind couldn't comprehend the depth and vastness of it.

On the other hand, I was taught that if people didn't believe in God in a very specific way, they would burn in hell forever. When I was young, my own mother wasn't very religious and I was afraid for her soul. I kept wondering, *How could a loving God threaten to put her in the fires of hell for all eternity?* I figured God must love my mother at least as much as I do, and I would never let that happen to her. It just didn't make any sense to me.

When I started working the steps with my sponsor, she told me I could redefine for myself what 'God' means. I was taken aback. I hadn't realized I could do that! The steps said that it was God as I understood it, so she helped me come up with a concept that made sense to me and that was how I was able to keep making progress with the steps.

The word that almost prevented me from gaining access to the program was just a symbol. By staying open-minded and curious, I found a treasure that had been there all long.

As I mentioned earlier, one of the ideas that changed my perspective early on was the concept of redefining those problematic words I was getting hung up on. There was a charismatic young woman at many of the meetings I attended. She was a thin, tall blonde who always looked like she was on her way to play softball. Her name was Mary. When she shared, her whole face lit up. She was so full of intensity and energy that she would draw you into her world and make you forget your surroundings. The way she could turn a phrase and touch my heart left me mesmerized. She'd been sober for over a year, and she openly shared that her thoughts on God had changed dramatically as she progressed through the steps.

She realized her concept of God had been passed down and reinforced by her parents when she was a child. When she'd first begun attending meetings, her sponsor said if she had a problem with God, she probably had a problem with someone else's God. That she could come up with her own concept of the Divine. That entire idea blew my mind! Yet, it made perfect sense to me. It gave me the hope I needed to keep going in the program, but with a definition I could build upon.

After all, I thought, *who gets to decide what God means to me...but me?*

But here's the thing: this book isn't going to be about me pointing at the metaphorical box you've been sitting on and pushing you to open it. I know from experience that when people push me, it creates internal resistance and makes me dig my heels in more deeply. I want you to think of this book more as an offering. Like we're hanging out, drinking coffee in my cozy living room. "This is what I used to think," I'd say, as I handed you a steaming mug, "then I learned this other way of looking at it, and this is how I integrated those ideas into my life. If you find an idea makes sense to you, you can incorporate it and keep moving forward. If not, keep seeking other perspectives until you find what works for you."

My recommendation is to trust the process, not necessarily the people—not even me. I learned a long time ago that I don't know what's right for anyone else. I also learned that we all have the answers inside of us. That's where the treasure lies. Although a good mentor will help you come to your own conclusions, the process itself will clear away the blocks to the truth that lies within you.

This book will include a transparent look into my own addictions and the program that started me on a lifelong journey of healing. A journey that has led to me becoming the best version of myself. It has changed the way I see the world and, more importantly, the way I see myself. The steps have revealed my true identity and that changed the way I live my life. There are examples of my personal experiences scattered throughout the book, as well as examples from others. After all, stories are what help us relate to one another. They help us see that if others can overcome addiction, we can too.

I believe I am somewhat unique in one aspect of my personality which is this odd desire to confront and resolve my character defects, even if it pisses me off at first. I learned that the truth might be painful, but it's also the thing that sets me free. By confronting painful truths about myself and accepting them, I am able to transcend them. Not only transcend them, but these truths can also be transformed into my superpowers because I will be able to use my experiences to help others.

For instance, I struggled with friendships for a long time. Making friends was not the problem, it was keeping them—but I didn't know why. With the help of my compassionate sponsor, I was able to see that I was often afraid of not getting my needs met, so my resulting behavior was often selfish and inconsiderate . I had such a desperate need to be seen, heard, and understood that I would often dominate conversations with my problems and not reciprocate. I was like an energy vampire. Everything was all about me. By accepting the truth, which was that I was treating my friends like unpaid therapists, I realized I was not being a good friend. Not only was I not giving back; I was also placing undue responsibility on others for my feelings, living in a constant state of disappointment and resentment. Through this process, I learned to take responsibility for my own feelings and add value to my friends' lives. I was finally able to make space for my friends to feel loved and supported.

The truth was that I didn't know how to meet my own needs or regulate my fears so that I could be a good friend to others. Over time, I developed the skills I needed to cultivate the deep and nurturing friendships I had always longed for. Skills like listening, showing empathy, taking an interest, and finding ways to make others feel important and cared for.

Looking back, I realize I was in deep denial. I had a victim mentality that kept me stuck in a cycle of suffering for a long time. What I know now is that I didn't have any healthy coping skills, so drinking was all I had to distract myself from the emotional pain I was carrying. I wasn't able to change until I hit an emotional rock-bottom. That's when I could no longer be in denial, and I began to see I had to give up blaming others and take full responsibility for myself.

Nowadays I am vigilant about not drifting back into a self-made mental prison through regular self-examination. Even though I do a lot of daily self-care, I know I still have blind spots. Thankfully, I have developed a strong support system of loving friends and talented professionals to help me identify and resolve my limiting beliefs as they arise.

I'm not alone in this quest for personal growth. There are millions of people out there seeking ways to heal. What I know for sure is that pushing people to see what they are not ready to experience creates even more resistance, which is the exact opposite of what I hope to accomplish with this book. But if you're sick and tired of feeling sick and tired—and you are ready to go to any lengths to change your life—you will find powerful tools and concepts that will help you to do the self-examination required for this profoundly transformational experience.

4

My Sober-Curious Crisis

To me, the term "sober curious" refers to the period when I started toying with the idea that I should quit drinking. It didn't happen until I was in a state of crisis.

My journey toward recovery began when I was 23 years old, after one of the worst nights of my life. Let me set the scene for you: I was just about ready to go out for the night. My hair and makeup were done, and af ter walking through a cloud of Giorgio perfume, I put on a new outfit I just bought. A sexy, black, off-the-shoulder sweater and a short floral skirt with black patent leather stiletto heels. I wanted to look as good as possible because I was going to be meeting up with Johnny, my ex-boyfriend's best friend, later that night at my favorite bar. This is the ex-boyfriend who also happened to be a married DUI cop. Yeah, I was that kind of girl.

Before I left my apartment, I wanted to get a little buzz going. I poured a tall water glass of red wine and proceeded to chug it down like medicine. Once the glass was drained, I felt the familiar warmth spread through my whole body. Now I was ready. I practiced this particular ritual nearly every time I went out. So much so that I had ceased feeling guilty about it. After all, drinking at home was cheaper, and I prided myself on being a very frugal party girl.

I got in my car and drove over to my mom's house to pick up my older sister, who was virtually the last friend I had. My other drinking buddies had turned into self-centered bitches seemingly overnight. To help bolster a false sense of confidence, I told myself I didn't care and that I was better off without them. Deep down, I knew that was far from the truth, but I wasn't going to let that stop me from having a good time.

The night began with the usual excitement and anticipation of a good time. We arrived at a packed bar, the sounds of loud music and laughter spilling out into the street. I pulled my sister across the smoke-filled room to the bar for a drink, a double vodka cranberry and soda. I'm pretty sure I had several in quick succession because that's what I always did, but the memories are a little hazy from that point on.

I remember laughing with some random people I just met and fawning over a guy I went to high school with but that's about it. What I don't remember is how I felt by the end of the night; my sister later told me I was furious because Johnny was a no-show—again. She told me I was ranting and raving about how he was probably with another woman and how jealous I was.

Bits of embarrassing moments from the evening still flash through my memory, like making out with the guy I'd gone to high school with. I vaguely remember how my sister was constantly straightening my off-the-shoulder sweater to keep me covered up and how she finally dragged me out of the bar to save me from humiliating myself even more.

This is where things took a turn for the worse because on the way home, we happened to pass my ex-boyfriend on the road, as he was giving a field sobriety test. Apparently, that was the last straw for me and it triggered an episode of drunken rage.

I don't remember most of this, but the next day my sister told me I'd completely lost my mind, punching the windshield with my fist a couple times, leaving large spiderweb-looking cracks on the passenger side. My sister told me that as she drove, I kept grabbing the wheel to crash the car. I also tried to jump out while she was still driving but she held onto my arm with her free hand.

We began fighting as she tried desperately to maintain control of the car. I then kicked her in the face, giving her a bloody nose. She managed to pull the car over in front of a friend's house and ran to their door for help as I screamed and sobbed in the middle of the street. The cops showed up and threatened to take me to jail if I didn't calm down. I have a brief memory of a woman telling me it wasn't worth it. I must have listened because I didn't go to jail that night.

Instead, I woke up the next morning back in my apartment. I was completely hung over, with a sickening, sinking feeling that something terrible had happened the night before. I could only remember bits and pieces of the evening and what I could remember was horrifying. Johnny was somehow in my bed sleeping peacefully like nothing happened, and my hand was swollen and purple. I didn't know how I hurt myself but somehow I wasn't that surprised. There were many mornings when I woke up with unexplained bruises or injuries.

That morning, I woke up with more questions than answers which wasn't that unusual, but something felt different this time. Somehow, I could sense I had reached a new low. Even after all this time, i t's hard to describe the gravity of the guilt, shame, and remorse I felt at that moment. The feelings of self-loathing and despair that washed over me that morning were almost unbearable. It all felt crushingly familiar—and I knew it had to stop.

As I lay there, I began wondering why I always got so drunk. Why had I let Johnny come over after he blew me off? Why had I lost my mind after I saw my ex on the way home? Why did I keep putting myself in these situations? What was wrong with me? I felt broken inside, and I was completely disgusted with myself. Again.

Johnny quickly disappeared, as usual, and I decided to go to my mother's house to talk to my sister and find out what happened. I received my first answer when I went downstairs and saw my car with the broken windshield. I thought, *So that's how I hurt my hand!* It felt like a punch to the gut. What a fucking loser…

When I arrived at my mom's house where my sister lived, she was so angry she could barely look at me. She was icy cold and scowling as she told me what had happened the night before. As she spoke, I felt my stomach sink as a fresh wave of shame, horror, and humiliation washed over me. It's not as if something crazy like this hadn't happened before but this was worse because I had involved my sister. I burned with shame knowing she had already told our mother the entire story.

Probably the oddest part about this conversation was when she mentioned she had decided to start attending Al-Anon meetings—a program for friends and family members of alcoholics. I remember my jaw dropped in shock and indignation as I gaped at her. I asked her, "You're going because of ME?!" I was in such denial about my drinking that I couldn't get over the fact that she thought I was an alcoholic. Looking back, it seems so painfully obvious.

That was the first time I stopped to consider that maybe she was right. It was the moment I became "sober curious," and started to ask myself all the questions I'd been avoiding for so long. *Am I really an alcoholic? What makes someone an alcoholic? What about all my friends who drank like I did? Were they alcoholics too? Have I crossed some invisible line? What if I really do have a problem? I can't fathom a life without drinking…*

One question led to another, but I didn't want the answer to be that I had to quit drinking for good. That was when I began an obsessive quest to figure out how to get control back and drink like a normal person.

So, in hopes of finding answers that didn't include abstinence I practically lived in the self-help section at Barnes & Noble. I spent hours poring over all the books that held answers to what I thought I wanted, to find Mr. Right and make lots of money. Surely if I was in love and had lots of money my life would be perfect, right? Since recovery memoirs weren't a thing yet in the 90s, I read books like *Men are from Mars, Women are From Venus*, and *The Seven Spiritual Laws of Success*. I read book after book looking for answers to all the wrong questions—all while trying to control my drinking.

This went on for two long and painful years. During that period, I tried to control my drinking on my own in a thousand different ways, always failing. I tried eating before I started drinking and downing a glass of water between drinks. I tried switching from mixed drinks to beer and wine. I tried to delay when I started drinking for the evening and limit the number of drinks I had. None of it worked. It seemed like as soon as that first drink slid down my throat, that feeling of wanting more kicked in and there was no telling how much I'd drink.

The morning after I'd wake up sick and tired, sometimes in strange places, and totally baffled as to how I ended up that way. I'd swear off drinking that morning once again, then forget how awful it had been by the evening, and I would start the process over again. It's not that I drank every day, but every time I drank, it was to excess—and I could never predict what would happen.

Those two years of trying to moderate my drinking were utterly exhausting, but now I know I had to do it. I had to go through that painful process of trial and error before I could completely surrender to the idea that I needed to practice abstinence and to accomplish it, I couldn't do it alone.

Truthfully, during that experimental period I didn't believe booze was the real issue. I suspected that deep down, there was something fundamentally wrong with me. I believed I was broken somehow and I needed to fix it, as every area of my life was a mess.

The irony is that I was so close to being right. Drinking *was* a symptom of a deeper problem, but I wasn't broken as a human being, I was deeply wounded without even realizing it, as I had completely dissociated from my painful experiences. I didn't know it at the time, but I had been living with unhealed trauma. Sexual abuse that I had endured when I was 5 years old at the hands of a neighbor. That was the core issue that needed to be addressed but I needed to be sober in order to deal with it.

Let me share a little story of a behavior pattern I indulged in over the years. I'd always thought of myself as a fun-loving party girl, searching for romantic love. My motto was, I'd try anything twice, just in case I didn't do it right the first time. I tried all kinds of drinks, lots of drugs, and dated all kinds of men. I would joke about my behavior by saying that if it was in a bottle, a bag, or blue jeans, I was doin' it! (and yes, that means what you think it means).

Friday would roll around and I'd get restless and lonely, so I'd go out with the girls to have some fun. It was exciting to get all dressed up, go out, and feel full of anticipation—but always with one thought in the back of my mind: Is this the night I finally meet 'the one'? Deep down, I was looking for love, but in all the wrong places.

So the girls and I would go out, get drinks, and we'd strut around, loving all the male attention. I was always searching for "him," my favorite kind of drug. But even if I *did* meet someone, and everything went right, there was always the inevitable disappointment that followed. Maybe I would get a little too drunk and repel someone I really liked, or maybe the guy I thought was a catch would end up revealing a flaw that repelled me. In either case, I would use alcohol to cope with the fallout of it all, and I would sink into a sea of self-loathing that left me mired in deep despair and self-hatred. By seeking to distract myself from emotional pain with drinking and seeking external validation, I was unknowingly creating the conditions that would cause even more pain—and I didn't even realize it.

While it is human nature to seek pleasure and avoid pain, addiction is about living in extremes . Looking back, I see that I created so much drama in my life just so I didn't have to be present to the pain of my trauma. That's how the brain works. It attempts to protect itself through dissociation and distraction, but that strategy doesn't work in the long term. The addictions themselves that begin as a coping mechanism eventually become more harmful than helpful.

Eventually, I ran out of ideas for controlling my drinking. I felt so defeated I finally surrendered to the idea that I couldn't drink like a normal person, and that's when I decided to tell my friend Mitch that I was ready to go to an AA meeting.

Truthfully, I thought my life was over. I felt a deep sense of loss and grief because I was losing the one thing that brought peace and joy into my life. I truly thought I'd never have any fun ever again. But to my surprise, a good life was just beginning. I was able to let go of the disappointing life I didn't even like anymore and build a new one on the firm, solid foundation of the 12 steps.

As I write this book, I have had continuous sobriety for over 30 years. I have been happily married to the love of my life since 1997, and we've raised two young men who have never had to see either of their parents drunk. While I'm obviously no saint, I am much closer to my authentic self than I was before I got sober.

My hope is that by hearing my story, and the way the program was taught to me and millions of others, you might gain the information you need to overcome any obstacles on your path to healing and wholeness. To have a transformational experience that feels nothing short of miraculous.

The 12 Steps: So What's the Big Deal?

At a high level, 12-Step programs are peer support groups founded on spiritual practices and principles, intended to help those struggling with addictions to overcome them. The program consists of meetings, its members, books, and the 12 steps and 12 traditions.

The steps are largely writing exercises assigned by a sponsor; someone who has previously worked the steps and acts as a mentor. Sponsors are typically not mental health professionals but members who share their experiences and suggestions with new members. They assume this role for many reasons. First, to pass along the information that helped them recover as a way to practice the 12th step. They also do it to help others quit drinking, as an act of service, to rebuild self-esteem, but also to maintain their own sobriety.

The 12 traditions are guidelines for the relationship between individual groups, the members, and the global community. They address issues of finance, public relations, and the overall purpose of the organization.

But the program is so much more than that. For me, it was a safe space. A place I'd often hear the experiences of other drinkers, what happened to them when they drank, and what life has been like since they quit. It was a place to make new friends, who understood the way I thought and felt, and where I could find a new normal. A place where I could share what was *really* going on in my life and still receive love and support.

I believe most people at meetings really try to speak from the heart. What I have come to understand is that the language of the heart crosses all boundaries and barriers. Simply put, pain recognizes pain. We might come from different backgrounds or look dissimilar from one another, or speak differently, but our underlying feelings are often the same. I would routinely see myself in others as they shared their stories, which was such a relief, as I thought I was the only one who'd felt that way. As my shame started to dissolve, my self-compassion grew.

For the first time in my life I felt seen, heard, and understood. I began to feel like I belonged somewhere, and I knew that I had found my people. In one of the first meetings I attended, "Welcome Home" was written on a chalkboard at the front of the room—and with those words, I knew I was home.

From my perspective, attending meetings has always been a matter of convenience as all the components I need for sobriety can be found in one place. In the early stages of my sobriety, I needed a safe space to make new friends; ones who didn't drink. I needed a place where I could review the principles of the program and hear how other members applied it to specific situations such as family, relationships, work, and society. Meetings are a place where I perform service work, which has been a great way to get to know people and rebuild my self-esteem.

Over time, I began to see that the program is simple, but not easy; and the fellowship as valuable, yet imperfect. Many ideas found therein can be confusing, and members who often struggle with mental health are known to debate every aspect of recovery and the literature. However, they also spend enormous amounts of time selflessly helping those who are suffering to honor the principles of the program, which is based on unity.

The goal of the 12-Step process is to help you gain access to a higher power, as you understand it, for guidance and strength. This higher power can help you to manage your emotions and lead a more peaceful, fulfilling life of purpose and meaning. One of the first things I was told when I began the program was that I needed to find a sufficient substitute for alcohol. For me that was the 12-Step program, a higher power, and a supportive community of likeminded individuals. I am deeply grateful for the people who have come before me and demonstrated a way of life that continues to benefit me to this day.

6

My 12-Step Adventure

Mitch and Randy were two clients I met through work back in 1993. They were kind and compassionate 12-Step members who shared their sobriety stories with me. They mentioned that they once drank like I did and couldn't stop, but they'd found a solution that had changed their lives.

Randy told me things that opened my mind to a new way of thinking, like that the definition of insanity was doing the same thing over and over and expecting a different result. For instance, I tried for a long time to control my drinking but nothing worked. I was still blacking out and making a complete ass of myself on a semi-regular basis. Randy pointed out that continuing to drink, after everything I had tried, was kind of insane. It was a little harsh, but he wasn't wrong. He told me that if I kept doing what I was doing, I'd keep getting what I was getting.

One day while sitting in Mitch's office, he gave me a little blue sheet of paper the size of a bookmark. It had a test on it to help the reader decide whether they had a problem with drinking. There were questions like, "Have you ever missed school or work due to drinking? Have you ever decided to stop drinking for a week or so, but only lasted for a couple of days? Have you ever switched from one kind of drink to another in the hope that this would keep you from getting drunk?"

To no one's surprise, I answered yes to every question. That's when Mitch first offered to take me a meeting, reassuring me that it was a free program—and that the only requirement for membership was a desire to stop drinking. He suggested that all I had to do was show up and listen before I made any decisions.

We decided to attend a meeting in a neighboring town, so I didn't have to run into anyone I knew. I was terrified. Thinking back to my first exposure to AA when I was 14, I asked him, "Are they going to introduce themselves by their first name and say they're an alcoholic?" He matter-of-factly said that they would. He also told me to listen for the similarities, not the differences. That way I would be able to identify the people I related to most, instead of looking for reasons why I didn't belong there.

After work one day, I got all dressed up and went with Mitch to this old strip mall where there was a room dedicated to meetings. My first impression was not great. The area was kind of dingy and run-down, and there was a group of sketchy people standing out front, smoking and talking. To say I felt awkward and self-conscious would be an understatement. We walked inside, past the clouds of cigarette smoke, and found seats at a table. In the corner was a table with coffee and cookies, something I'd grow accustomed to seeing at almost every meeting I attended thereafter. There was also a rack of pamphlets and display books. Mitch bought me a blue "Big Book," which is really titled *Alcoholics Anonymous*.

It was comforting to have some moral support from Mitch and a buffer to a bunch of strangers. Some members were clearly hard-luck cases and looked a little rough around the edges, but there were also many professional people who looked like Mitch and Randy. There were a few well-dressed women in the room, and I remember feeling surprised that they had a problem with alcohol, too.

When the meeting started, the secretary welcomed all the newcomers. I felt like I was sitting in the middle of a spotlight because everyone turned to look at me as the obvious new person. Then came the moment I'd been dreading when they asked if anyone was there for the first time or in their first 30 days. I blurted out my name, and choked on the word, "alcoholic." Everyone smiled and clapped, welcoming me. I felt incredibly relieved when that part was over.

Next, she asked if anyone was celebrating a milestone of sobriety. A lot of 12-Step meetings offer medallions or "chips" marking periods of sobriety.

A guy stood up, said his name, and that he had been sober for 30 days. He looked to be in his 30s, wearing a white T-shirt and baggy pants and he was covered in tattoos. He looked like he'd just gotten out of jail, but he was smiling and put his hand over his heart in a gesture of gratitude. Everyone clapped as he walked up to the front of the room. The secretary handed him a 30-day chip and gave him a hug. A few others did this announcing various milestones. A nicely dressed lady had two years, an older man in a business suit had seven years, and a man with a black leather biker vest claimed 14 years! I didn't even know these people, but I felt so happy for them. I was even starting to feel a glimmer of hope for myself.

From there, my memory is a bit of a blur. I don't remember what anyone said, but I do remember feeling like I was home. People were saying all the things I'd secretly felt: they'd never felt as if they fit in anywhere before. Or they had been carrying painful feelings of guilt and shame for things they had done.

They said things out loud that shocked me—not because of their content, but because they were so open about them. Before attending my first meeting, there were things I swore I'd never say out loud. But as I watched the other members recount their stories so casually, I started to think maybe there was something to this whole open, honest, and vulnerable thing. For instance, if you struggle with alcohol apparently it's normal to wake up from a blackout not knowing where you are or how you got there. One woman joked about how that was a common occurrence for her! In my head I was screaming, "Oh my God, shut up! They're all going to judge you!" But everyone would just laugh knowingly. No one clutched their pearls in shock.

The stories I heard in that room were tragic; inspiring; and even hilarious, at times. I'd never heard people talk in such an open and transparent way before. For the first time in my life, I felt there were people in the world who understood me. Driving home after that first meeting, I had hope that I had finally found a place where I belonged.

As I attended more meetings, I quickly learned that my preconceived ideas about the other members were totally wrong. They were doctors, lawyers, teachers, construction workers, stay-at-home parents, preachers, nuns—people from all walks of life. There was every race present, not to mention all ages, sexes, and spiritual beliefs or no spiritual beliefs at all.

The fact is that alcohol is accepted in nearly every culture, and it is physically and mentally addictive. If you combine that fact with underlying trauma, mental health issues, and a lack of coping skills, you have a recipe for disaster that does not discriminate.

My fears about who those people at meetings would be were largely unfounded. Due to the nature of the program members often hold service positions. The program teaches us that to stay sober members should attend meetings regularly, help run them by accepting service positions, contribute financially when they can, and share their experiences of how they got sober. Service helps rebuild your self-esteem and allows you to feel part of a group, which is important as so many of us feel we've never fit in anywhere at all.

To "work the program" means to read the literature, work the steps with your sponsor, carry the message of recovery to the newcomers, and live by the program's principles. Very early on, I heard that I should do 90 meetings in 90 days. That I should find a female sponsor who had what I wanted, to take me through the steps. The thought of that was terrifying! Up until then, I didn't have good relationships with women. I mostly saw them as competition for male attention. But I was so desperate to stay sober that I decided to look for a sponsor.

As I went to meetings, women would go out of their way to welcome me or offer me their phone numbers. They would offer suggestions like, "watch out for wolves in sheep's clothing," indicating that some of the men might ask me out on a date, and that I should stay focused on getting healthier and not look for romance. One lady suggested that I try to avoid relationships for the first year—which sounded outrageous—until she told me, "Water seeks its own level," meaning if I wasn't healthy yet, I would attract an unhealthy partner as well.

There was also a lot of talk about the ominous 4th step. I kept hearing about people who would do Steps 1-3, then relapse, and have to start over. I was so scared of drinking again that I decided to ask a woman to sponsor me. You know how I picked her? She remembered my name the second time she met me. It was as if the clouds parted and brilliant rays of sunshine illuminated her, as if she were an angel. And you know how I asked her to be my sponsor? I asked if she would be willing to listen to my 4th step. I'll never forget what she said next. She stopped in her tracks, looked me in the eye and with such gentleness said, "I'd be honored." To this day the memory of that moment makes me want to cry. Then she said, "But we're going to start at Step 1." Her name was Kimmerz, and I'll be forever grateful to her.

Kimmerz was about my age and had already been sober for two years. When she got up to share, I was always touched by what she said. I was so impressed with her ability to be vulnerable and honest about how she was feeling and what she was learning about herself through the steps.

After she agreed to sponsor me, she suggested a time and place to meet to talk about the process. Kimmerz said we would read the book together and then she would give me a homework assignment and a deadline. She made it clear that if I didn't complete the homework before the deadline, we would reschedule. She explained that her role was to take me through the steps the way she had done them, to be honest with me about what had come up for her as she listened, and that she would share her experience, but not give me advice.

She had such good boundaries that I was a little intimidated by her at first. But because she had those firm boundaries, I understood what was expected of me, what I could expect of her, and it became the foundation of my first healthy relationship with another woman.

The following includes the steps, the principle behind each one, the homework assignments Kimmerz gave me, and my experiences as I went through them.

Step 1: "We admitted we were powerless over alcohol—that our lives had become unmanageable."

Interpretation: I came to realize I was powerless over alcohol, and I learned all the ways that drinking made my life unmanageable.

Principle: Honesty

We started with Step 1. My homework was to write out the dictionary definitions of the words "powerless" and "unmanageable." Then I had to think about my past, giving examples of how or when I was *powerless over alcohol*, which wasn't hard. There were so many examples to choose from. The most obvious being that I was powerless over how much I drank once I started. I never intended to black out when I drank, but I did black out quite a bit.

For instance, one night my boss—who loved to drink as much as I did—had me meet him and a couple of our clients at a nice restaurant with a bar. Everything started out fine. I remember showing up in my fancy business suit, looking classy and professional. There was a lot of champagne, and we were talking and laughing, having a good time. That's all I remember. I woke up the next morning at home with a terrible hangover and spent the entire morning vomiting violently, which happened almost every time I blacked out. It was alcohol poisoning. I didn't even realize that's what it was because it happened so often; I just thought that's what a normal hangover was.

The next evening, I went back to the same bar to meet my boss again. By the bartender's reaction the moment I walked in, I could tell something had happened between us the previous night. He was way too happy to see me and I had no idea why. I could tell he was offended that I wasn't as happy to see him which was super awkward. Did I treat him like my new BFF? Did I make out with him? Who knows. But it wasn't cool. Especially since I had a boyfriend at the time. I felt horrible about myself.

Another way I knew I was powerless over alcohol was that once I started drinking, I never knew which of my multiple personalities was going to emerge. My behavior was totally unpredictable—even to me.

Sometimes when I started drinking, the feelings of wanting more would kick into overdrive. It didn't happen every time I drank, but I had no control over when it would get triggered. On the nights it did, I got into a lot of trouble. The kind that involves pointless arguments with friends, and guys I dated, and occasionally the police. I never got arrested or went to jail, but I lost nearly all my friends toward the end of my drinking. Not so surprisingly, I didn't have any romantic relationships that survived past my drunken episodes. I didn't get into trouble every time I drank, but every time I got into trouble it was when I had been drinking. So, yeah, it became clear that I was powerless over alcohol.

Kimmerz also asked me to think about the ways my life was unmanageable due to alcohol. No problem. Clearly I was not managing my life very well, considering I had ruined all my relationships and my finances were a mess. Not to mention I usually didn't know how I got home after I drank—if I made it home at all. There were nights I'd drive with one eye closed, as I was seeing double. It's horrifying to think of what could have happened. I was incredibly lucky that I didn't kill myself—or anyone else.

This exercise from Step 1 helped me to see both the gravity and reality of my relationship with alcohol. I wrote down many examples of unmanageability that I was deeply ashamed of. Seeing it on the page in black and white stripped me of any denial about my drinking and gave me the motivation I needed to practice abstinence.

Part of Step 1 was to read the list out loud to Kimmerz, which was incredibly uncomfortable but I was so desperate to be sober that I did it. She shared stories of similar things she did too which gave me courage to continue. You know, not once did I catch a glimmer of judgment in her eyes as I shared my experiences with her. Not once did she flinch or look at me sideways. I could see in her eyes that she understood my kind of crazy. She told me I never had to drink again if I didn't want to and I believed her. Throughout this process, she expressed nothing but compassion and empathy. She knew I didn't want to be this way. She understood I was suffering from alcoholism.

It was probably the first real experience of intimacy I ever had. I let her see who I really was and she didn't reject me. On the contrary, she offered me love and acceptance. That feeling of being lost and alone that I'd carried around my entire life began to evaporate on the spot. It was revolutionary.

Step 2: "Came to believe that a power greater than ourselves could restore us to sanity."

Interpretation: I came to understand that spirituality could help me heal in ways that I couldn't heal alone and think more objectively.

Principle: Hope

Through this step, I was able to make a fresh start with a higher power that made sense to me in the hopes of receiving help to live a purposeful and productive life.

Although I grew up in a Christian home, attending church every Sunday, I didn't grow up having a healthy relationship with God.

Looking back, I felt resentful that God didn't protect me from the sexual abuse I endured starting at age 5 which lasted for several years. Those experiences left me feeling dirty, guilty, and ashamed of myself. After my parents divorced when I was seven, I thought it was my fault. If only I had been good enough, they wouldn't have split up.

When I was in my early teens, I really wanted to be a good girl. We went to church a couple times per week and I loved God. I wanted to do the things that were expected of me, like do what I'm told, be kind, get good grades, and get along with my sister but I always fell short. I also knew I had to stop doing the things I knew were wrong. I was already sneaking out with my friends, meeting up with boys, and experimenting with drugs and alcohol. It was like I just couldn't stop myself from being bad.

I would beg God to help me be good but no matter how hard I prayed to be strong, I felt weak. I would give into temptation and I failed again and again. At some point, I just gave up. I decided that if I couldn't be good, I was going to be good at being bad.

But I was still expected to go to church.

In high school I became good friends with the pastor's daughter. She was tall, beautiful, and a pothead. She said she smoked weed so often that NOT being high was her altered reality. When she said that, it hit me like a ton of bricks—that's what I wanted. She was my hero. I did everything in my power to hang out with her and to be just like her. Being high on weed was my favorite thing in the world. It was so much fun; I loved the feeling of being numb.

It was such a confusing time. I was completely conflicted about God. On one hand, I had experiences that felt like God's love. Sometimes the music at church was so emotional and powerful that feelings of love would wash over me, touching the deepest parts of my heart. I would pray when I was sad and hurting from all my self-hatred, and it felt comforting to think there was a God that forgave me for my sins and truly loved me.

However, even though I had been baptized as a baby, was saved at a Billy Graham crusade when I was 14, and even got dunked at the Baptist church, I was pretty sure my soul was still in jeopardy. I had always felt bad inside and knew I couldn't hide who I was from God.

After my parents' divorce my older sister and I lived with my mom. Dad lived close by, and he was the gentler, more nurturing one of the two. My mom was not. She had two predominant feelings when I was growing up: either really happy or really pissed—and I felt like she saved her happy face for the outside world. She could be screaming at me for not cleaning the house one minute and then flip like a switch to being happy and cheerful when her friends called.

This left me with two predominant feelings too: guilty and wrong.

To be fair, my mother often worked long hours at a stressful corporate job. She must have been exhausted when she got home only to find it a mess, which drove her insane. I remember the feeling of sheer panic I felt each time I heard her car pull into the driveway. She would walk in, take one look around the house, and then rage at us for not cleaning up after ourselves. There was never any resolution or absolution afterward. I just bottled up all my feelings that eventually turned into self-hatred.

So, one night when I was around 9 years old, I got drunk for the first time.

My mom was out on a dinner date, leaving me and my older sister home alone. I'm not sure where I got the idea to drink, but that night I found a dusty old bottle of booze in the cabinet. I never saw my parents drink so I don't know how it got there, but I thought it would be fun to try it. My sister wasn't interested—being the good, compliant child—so it was a party of one!

I'll never forget that first fumy sip of booze mixed with juice. It tasted awful. It burned my lips, burned all the way down, but when it hit bottom, a feeling of warmth spread through my entire body. I hadn't realized how bad I had always felt until suddenly I felt really good. It was as if all my fear, guilt, shame, and self-loathing had been lifted, and all that was left was this amazing, warm, buzzy feeling. I went from anxious to bliss in just a few disgusting swallows. The juxtaposition of those two feelings was so intense it was burned into my psyche forever. I had gone from hating who I was to feeling completely happy and free. It was that feeling of relief that I would chase for years to come.

Of course, I didn't become a regular binge drinker at that point. It was years later when I was 14 that I started to drink more regularly. In junior high I would even sometimes drink before school. Mostly I would drink on the weekends with my friends when we could sneak it in at a sleepover. All this was going on while still going to church on Sundays and youth groups on Wednesdays. Even though I wanted to be good, I loved to drink and get high and I was completely boy crazy. Apparently, no amount of begging God to fix me was going to change all of that so I eventually gave up on God.

By the time I was 25, my drinking was so out of control I knew I had to quit for good. It was the morning after my birthday celebration, yet another night of blackout drinking where I'd totally humiliated myself in front of my boyfriend and friends. I had spent all morning with my head in the toilet, when I finally flopped onto the couch, looked at my boyfriend and told him, "I'm never drinking again." And I hadn't. But as soon as those words left my lips, I took a big bong hit to kill the nausea. Back in the day, they called it the "marijuana maintenance" program, and I was on it for five months until I started going to 12-Step meetings—which I soon learned is a program of total abstinence.

I shared all this with Kimmerz. She explained that in Step 3, "as we understood him," meant that I could design a concept of God that made sense to me. She told me it didn't even have to be a "him".

She asked me to write two columns on a piece of paper. One column was what God isn't; the other side, what God is. On the "isn't" side, I wrote words like "judgmental," "punishing," "cruel," "disinterested," and on the "is" side, I wrote things like "Has no gender," "loves me unconditionally," "is forgiving," "is all-knowing and all powerful," "is the master organizer and planner," "not restricted by time or space."

I read the lists to Kimmerz and then she asked for the page so I handed it to her. She literally tore it in half and handed me back the "God is" side and said, "If this is what you understand, this is your concept of a higher power and we're going to burn the other half." I was stunned. I was like, you can DO that?? She said we could, that it's what she had done, and it was working for her. Kimmerz told me that my concept would grow and evolve over time and that was okay.

Kimmerz also helped me to understand that the "came to believe" part was a process I would reach through my experiences, that would translate into evidence. By attending meetings, I was seeing the process work for others who were once where I was, who had worked the steps and were staying sober by relying on a higher power. They had to take responsibility and do the work, but by asking for help they were staying sober and living productive lives. As the days and weeks went by, I did come to believe there WAS a power greater than myself.

As I attended more meetings, I often heard people talk about what was working for them. One guy said he thought of God like "The Force" from *Star Wars*. A popular author, Carolyn Myss, gave her concept of God as Universal Law, but it was also personal to her. It was a presence that loved and cared for her personally, as it did everyone. That is an idea that has continued to make sense to me throughout my journey. I've also heard GOD described as an acronym for the phrase, "Group of Drunks," to represent the combined power of the group. Still others feel connected to a higher power in nature or the "Great Outdoors." All these concepts speak to the idea that you're not alone—that there is help available.

The "restore us to sanity" part was interesting. Clearly, I had not behaved sanely if I was blacking out, putting myself in harm's way, or unable to maintain healthy relationships. *Was I ever sane*, I wondered? *Was there ever a time when I wasn't full of fear or confusion?* I wasn't sure but I knew I wanted to reach a place where I felt in control of my emotions and my actions were in alignment with my values, and who I wanted to be. All my life I had been trying to get what I thought I wanted, to be who I thought I should be—and failing miserably in the process. But now there was a glimmer of hope. Maybe there *was* a power greater than myself and through it I would be restored to sanity.

By working Step 2 I learned I had been doing the same thing over and over, expecting a different result. I had the evidence and experience to prove that trying to control my drinking didn't work. I also had the evidence and experience to prove that I couldn't do it alone.

Help would come in the form of people. It seemed to me that God was working in my life through people like Mitch, Randy, and now Kimmerz. There were countless other people I saw at meetings that I was beginning to get to know better who were demonstrating that they were being restored to sanity.

Step 3: "Made a decision to turn our will and our lives over to the care of God as we understood him."

Interpretation: Having a basic understanding of a loving higher power I could trust, I decided to be open to receiving guidance in all areas of my life.

Principle: Surrender

Once I had a concept of God that made sense to me, it was time to turn my will and my life over into God's care. I kept hearing people at meetings say things like "surrender to win" but I didn't get it.

Together Kimmerz and I read Step 3 in both *Twelve Steps and Twelve Traditions* and in *Alcoholics Anonymous* so I could get a better understanding of it.

The literature talks about how we try to play God, but I didn't see it that way. In my mind I was trying to take responsibility for my happiness by doing what I thought I should do to get what I wanted. What I started to see was that I was full of fear. Fear that I wasn't going to get what I wanted or fear that I was going to lose something I already had. When I am fearful, I am tempted to act in ways that are self-centered, controlling, and manipulative. I had lots of evidence already that having fearful thoughts led to making fearful decisions, which led to fearful actions that did not have positive outcomes.

This is how I became willing to consider turning my will and my life over to the care of God.

Kimmerz and I talked about how to apply this principle of surrendering my will and asking for God's Will. She suggested that when a challenging situation came up, to pause for a moment and ask God for guidance. To be open to the highest and greatest good for all involved and trust my higher power to reveal a peaceful path forward.

There were many opportunities to practice this at work.

At the time I was working in a tuxedo shop. There was a situation where a party of seven groomsmen were returning their tuxedos, but because they were unhappy about something they decided to ball up all the clothes, cuff links, ties, and shoes into the bottom of the garment bags. It was a huge mess. The shop was full of people and I was the only one there at the time. I was afraid of these guys because they were clearly trying to make me uncomfortable, which triggered rage inside me.

I figured this would be a good time to practice surrendering. So I paused, took a deep breath, and asked God for guidance and strength. I asked for the highest and greatest good for all involved even though I felt very angry. In a calm voice, I told them they'd have to wait until I was done helping the other customers because of the condition of the returns. That they could leave, but if anything was missing, it would be charged to their credit cards. They waited.

After helping everyone else, I calmly went through all their returns. I didn't have an attitude, I spoke calmly and worked quickly to get them out. As I was going through everything, my co-worker Sam showed up to help me. She actually knew one of the guys! The whole mood lightened when they greeted each other. She gave her friend a hard time about the returns, and he clearly felt bad. He told her that they were all hung over and upset that they had to bring the tuxedos back so soon.

After they left Sam and I talked about what happened before she got there. She said how impressed she was with how I handled the situation. In that moment I realized what it looked like from the outside. She didn't know how angry I felt on the inside; all she saw was that I was calm. In the past I know I would have handled that differently. I would have been rude back to them, said some things that were unprofessional, and made the situation ten times worse. But I asked God for help and help literally came in the form of Sam—and just in the nick of time.

By practicing Step 3, I had evidence that help came in that situation and it gave me the incentive to keep asking for help in future challenging situations.

Kimmerz and I completed Step 3 by praying together. We got on our knees, held hands, and I said the Step 3 prayer right out of Page 63 of *Alcoholics Anonymous*. "God, I offer myself to thee — to build with me and **to** do with me as Thou wilt. Relieve me of the bondage of self, that I may better do Thy will. Take away my difficulties, that victory over them may bear witness to those I would help of Thy power, Thy Love, and Thy Way of life. May I do Thy will always!"

Step 4: "Made a searching and fearless moral inventory of ourselves."

Interpretation: Completed an honest yet compassionate self-examination writing exercise to uncover the root causes of my mental and emotional pain.

Principle: Courage

When I showed up to the program, I was completely self-centered yet incapable of self-examination. My life was a mess and I didn't know how to fix it. It was explained to me that Step 4 is a self-examination exercise designed to help you sort through all your pain, resolve resentments, and gain clarity to see where you can take personal responsibility and let go of burdens that were never yours to carry. This is where the magic happened for me.

Kimmerz and I read *Alcoholics Anonymous* together and she showed me the example on Page 70 of how to do the writing exercise. She held up a piece of notebook paper sideways and folded it into 4 columns, titling each column just as in the example. The first column was a list of people I was resentful toward, the second was the specific cause of my resentment, the third was how I was affected by the resentment, and the fourth column detailed my role in the interaction.

Even though the entire reason I'd asked her to be my sponsor was to do this step, it was still incredibly difficult. We had been meeting about once a week to go over my step work, but this step was taking much longer than I expected. It was hard to force myself to sit down, pen in hand, and dredge up all my painful resentments. Even more difficult to think about the specific causes of my resentments. But I was desperate to stay sober, so I leaned into it.

The resentment list started with my family. When I was growing up, my mom, sister, and I would get into the craziest arguments over the most minor infractions. It was usually over chores we didn't finish while our mom was at work. She would come home after a stressful day and be furious about the messy house and would want to know who to blame. Of course, my sister and I would blame each other which just pissed her off even more.

When her rage was directed at me she would bring up everything I'd ever done wrong in my entire life. First, it was that I didn't clean something the exact way she told me to—there was a way to do things and her way was the only way. Then it was my grades and how that time I lost my retainer. How I never did what I was told, or how I was always lazy. Pretty soon there were 10 things on the table I was being accused of. After a while I could no longer keep track of what we were even arguing about. I remember defending myself, blaming my sister while she was doing the exact same thing to me—both of us out of survival. There was a lot of denial going on too. It was a common practice to deny any responsibility for hurtful things that were done or said by repeating phrases like, "I never said that" or "I never did that." It was all very crazy-making.

Obviously nothing was ever resolved but everyone was hurt and angry. I can't even remember how the arguments would end, but eventually we'd all storm off to our separate rooms, crying and screaming at each other as we left. Mom would turn into a dictator, laying down harsh rules and saying things like, "From now on, this is how things are going to be done or else!" I would sit in my room, filled with rage and no way to process it. I remember feeling like a caged animal, wanting desperately to leave my room but having nowhere to go. I hated living there. In those moments, I hated both of them.

But things would slowly quiet down, I'd eventually fall asleep, and the next morning always held a special kind of tension in the air. It was so thick you could cut it with a knife. If I was lucky, Mom would have already left for work. I could maneuver around my sister because she was weak and if she said anything to me, I could easily shut her down. Most of the time she avoided me just as much as I avoided her.

Nothing was ever resolved but time would pass—along with our anger—and we'd test the waters with trivial comments once again. Sometimes, depending on her mood, my mom would act like nothing had happened, especially if she knew she'd taken things too far. I often look back and think about how hard it must have been for her to be working full time with all the stress that comes with it, only to come home to a messy house. I suspect she was so stressed out that just seeing dirty dishes in the sink was enough to push her over the edge and that her rage was merely misdirected.

She was probably venting because she never learned any healthy coping skills. But I didn't have any of that context at the time. The message I got was that I wasn't good enough and that her anger was my fault. These feelings were reinforced over and over again for years.

Looking back, it was no wonder I felt the need to find an escape from my feelings.

It was hard to look at those resentments and try to get specific about the cause. I'd call Kimmerz and explain it, so she could help me sort it all out. She would ask me questions like, "Would you say one of the causes was that she yelled at you for not cleaning up before she got home?" I'd answer yeah, absolutely! She'd ask how that affected me. Did it hurt my self-esteem, emotional security, and my personal relationship with her? I was like, *Hell yeah—it did all that!* Then she asked the tough question: for me to describe my part in that one specific situation. Before I knew it, I was feeling super defensive. "I was just a kid," I stammered, "She didn't have to yell at me like that or say all those hurtful things!"

Kimmerz would validate my feelings by agreeing with me, but she'd gently say, "That is true and I could see how you'd feel that way—but this is your inventory, not hers. Your job is to simply look at your part and consider how your behavior might have affected others." There was something about her gentleness that leveled my pride. I felt safe around her, and I trusted her because of my experience working through the first three steps together. She told me if I wanted to stay sober, I needed to be free of my past and that to resolve it, I needed to face it. So I did.

Kimmerz suggested I do a brain dump, and just start with a list of people I was resentful toward. I wrote down the names of family members, guys I dated, and friends I had lost. I listed former employers and random strangers—anyone I held negative feelings toward. Once I had my list, I went back to the top and addressed one person at a time. I wrote all the specific causes for that person and all the ways I was affected.

For instance, I listed a friend I had lost and the specific reasons I was resentful toward her. One of the worst resentments was how she made fun of me in front of a guy I liked. It was humiliating and left me feeling angry and helpless to defend myself. This affected my self-esteem and sense of emotional security, not to mention my personal relationship with her.

And what was my part? Well, the truth was she and I had a very toxic relationship. We did things to hurt each other all the time. If I was angry with her, I wouldn't speak to her directly. I'd stuff my feelings deep inside, then lash out in a passive-aggressive way later. She did the same to me. As it related to my resentment, I may have even provoked her but she and I had gone back and forth in this way for so long I didn't remember who started things.

Another way I was responsible in this situation is that I chose to be around her. I knew she had a wicked sense of humor and a way of being cruel, but I kept hanging out with her because I didn't want to be alone. I learned that I needed to take responsibility for my part in our toxic relationship and recognize that I hurt her too; that I used her as much as she'd been using me.

By the time I was done writing my whole 4th step there were pages and pages of resentments. As I wrote, repeating patterns began to emerge. I saw myself clearly for the first time. How I treated people, how I blamed people for how they made me feel, how I was overly dependent on some, and how I tried to control others.

One of the patterns I saw right away was that I often took responsibility for the feelings of others—but not for my own. When I was in my early teens, my older sister suffered from depression. It was painful to watch her suffer and since I loved her I tried to take responsibility for her feelings and make her feel better.

My mom modeled this behavior too. My sister never quite fit in anywhere and she had been intermittently bullied in elementary and middle school. We didn't have a lot of money, but to try to help her fit in Mom would take her to fancy salons to manage her super curly hair. Then she'd take her to the mall to get her makeup done professionally and buy all the products for her.

None of our efforts had much of an effect on my sister's depression and by the time she was in high school, she had reached a point of crisis.

Mom pulled me aside one day, looking worried in a way I'd never seen before. She was never afraid of anything, so her vulnerability completely shook me. She told me we had to stay close to my sister, and to keep an eye on her.

For as long as I could remember, even though it may not have been true, I felt that my mom had disdain for me. She didn't really "get" me as a person. In fact, she would literally say, "I don't understand you" so it wasn't my imagination. But in this moment, I felt like she needed me. I was determined not to let her down. I was going to save my sister.

Being the rescuer was like being on a rollercoaster that carried my peace with it. If my sister was grateful or happy for my efforts, I was at peace. If she suffered, I felt like a failure and was wracked with guilt and shame. To avoid those feelings, I would try even harder by offering unsolicited advice. When that didn't work, I'd become frustrated and resort to more assertive and controlling tactics. I would pepper her with questions intended to force her to see the error of her ways. I would always end up feeling resentful toward her for not changing. It's no surprise that she felt resentful toward me too.

Writing out the 4th step is how I learned about my deep-seated need to rescue others. That need to rescue is burned so deep into my psyche that I still need to be mindful of my motives when helping others to this day. It often shows up in the form of unhealthy friendships that mirror the relationship I had with my sister.

The 4th step revealed some limiting beliefs I had. Deep down, I believed if I saved my sister my mother would love me the way I wanted her to. It turned out to be a setup for the repeated experience of failure on my part.

I listed my specific resentments toward my sister: she wouldn't take any of the actions required to improve her condition, and it caused me pain and frustration to see her suffer. Consequently, it affected my self-esteem as I felt I was failing her. It also affected my emotional security because the repeated pattern caused feelings of guilt and shame.

When it came to my part, it was fairly obvious to me that I was taking inappropriate responsibility for her feelings without taking responsibility for my own. I had been prideful to think I knew what was right for her, or that I could save her. I indulged in self-righteous anger and I'd punish her with ridicule when she wouldn't change her behavior or take responsibility for her own feelings.

In a way, I was making her responsible for *my* feelings. As long as I needed her to be different so I could be okay, I was giving her power over my emotions. That realization hit me like a ton of bricks. I started to recognize a similar pattern in many of my other relationships too!

It wasn't until I did the 4th step that I saw these patterns were driven by self-centered fear. That my motives were not clean. I wasn't helping my sister end her suffering. I wanted her to stop suffering to ease my own pain.

The rest of my resentments followed a similar pattern. Someone did me wrong, and my self-esteem took hit after hit until there was nothing left. No wonder I carried so much guilt, shame, and self-loathing. My motives were not hard to identify. My actions were self-centered; I wanted other people to be responsible for my feelings.

Kimmerz and I also did the sex conduct inventory and a fears inventory. Although it was just more of the same, what was different about the sex conduct was that I saw how I used men like a drug. Every encounter followed a similar pattern. I would choose emotionally unavailable men, hang all my hopes and dreams on them, and waste hours thinking about them—only to feel disappointed and full of self-pity in the end.

What I learned about myself is that I had such low self-esteem that stemmed from my childhood trauma. Deep down I didn't believe I deserved anything better. In fact I hated who I was, so true intimacy was terrifying to me. Seeking emotionally unavailable men was a way to make someone else responsible for my feelings, with no hope of ever being happy. I learned this kind of love addiction was a distraction from my pain. If I indulged in romantic fantasies, I wasn't in the present moment which was intolerable. But there was a price to pay for that kind of indulgence. I would end up with even lower self-esteem and go into a very dark place of self-hatred. For this reason, I believe love addiction can be just as devastating as any other form of addiction.

The last part of the inventory was to write out a list of my fears, and how those fears had driven my actions up until this point. Most of them boiled down to fear of losing something I had, or fear of not getting what I wanted. When we dug deeper, I saw that those fears came from the fact that I didn't believe I could trust my higher power for help and therefore I had to be self-reliant. Always.

For me the 4th step was a process of revealing the facts. For breaking through the self-denial that had been keeping me stuck in a victim mentality for years. I had been walking around believing I was a victim of life; this exercise helped me to see I had a part in every resentment I held and that I could take back my power by recognizing where I made disempowering choices. It freed me from self-pity, self-centeredness, and self-sabotaging behaviors. It continues to be a useful exercise that allows me to see where I can evolve in a healthy way, without guilt or shame.

Step 5: "Admitted to God, to ourselves, and to another human being the exact nature of our wrongs."

Interpretation: After gaining clarity about my motives and behavior from step 4, I share what I learned about myself with someone else.

Principle: Integrity

With the writing finally finished, I made an appointment to meet with Kimmerz to share it. We had been talking throughout the writing process, so I wasn't too nervous, but she said it would probably take all day to go through it in detail. When I arrived at her apartment, we said a prayer for guidance before we began.

She took out a pad of paper and listed out the 7 deadly sins: Pride, Greed, Lust, Envy, Jealousy, Sloth, and Wrath. She said she would be listening for these in what I shared and would be making tally marks so that we could identify patterns. She explained that my instincts to get my needs met were normal but that out of balance they were character defects. This concept is spelled out clearly in both *Alcoholics Anonymous*, along with *The Twelve Steps and Twelve Traditions* which we had read together prior to writing out the inventory.

I read her the name of every person I was resentful toward, the exact cause, how I was affected and then, my part in the situation. There were some instances where I struggled to identify my part, like when I was sexually abused as a little girl. I was clear about the cause of my resentment, and how it affected me, but I didn't see what my part had been. Obviously, I was not responsible for what happened to me. It was not my fault, but what we did talk about was what I had done thus far as an adult to heal from it.

I hadn't done anything. No therapy or counseling to address it at all. Honestly, it hadn't even occurred to me to get help because I was so disassociated from the pain of those early childhood experiences that I was in complete denial of them. I was in survival mode. That's what early childhood trauma does; it makes you believe there isn't even a problem to solve. I had no frame of reference, so I didn't know what had happened to me wasn't normal. I just felt like it was my fault.

Kimmerz helped me to understand that unresolved pain shows up in seemingly unrelated ways. I just decided at some point that I wasn't a good person, or that I wasn't good enough to be happy. That was probably why I settled for emotionally unavailable partners or abusive friendships. My deep, subconscious beliefs were that I didn't deserve anything better. It wasn't until we started examining how my self-esteem was damaged repeatedly that I had concluded I wasn't a good person. It was a belief that was so integrated into my identity I didn't even know where it had come from. That's when my part in the situation became clear. I'd felt like a victim for my entire life, and I was stuck in that mentality. I realized in that moment that what had happened to me wasn't my fault, but my happiness and well-being *was* my responsibility. Nobody was going to rescue me; I had to do the work myself. That's when I decided to get professional help—and that's when I started to heal from the abuse.

We went over all my resentments. I saw that I was self-centered, only thinking about what I wanted or how I felt. That's how I was showing up in all my relationships. It was painful to acknowledge the truth but that's where I found freedom.

I was lucky to have a good sponsor in Kimmerz. She validated my feelings by saying things like, "Yeah, I could see how you'd feel that way," or "I was like that, too." As she told her stories, it gave me the courage to share more of mine, the resentments I held toward guys I had dated, friends I had lost, the people I hurt...all of it.

She had been keeping a tally of character defects, and it was no surprise that pride was my biggest one. There were tally marks for every deadly sin but strangely I didn't feel bad when I was done—quite the opposite. I felt a huge relief, a high, like when I'd taken my first drink. I had faced my past, received clarity on where I was out of balance, and the guilt and shame had been lifted—leaving me feeling euphoric.

Kimmerz told me to go home and reflect on our time together, just as the book suggests. By the time I got home I was emotionally exhausted and slept for hours. I knew there were people I was going to have to make amends to, but she said we weren't quite there yet. I needed to do a few more steps first to gain clarity but, together, we would get there.

Step 6: "Were entirely ready to have God remove all these defects of character."

Interpretation: With self-compassion and an understanding of what drives my negative behavior, I ask my higher power to help me heal and make different choices.

Principle: Willingness

For this step, Kimmerz and I read aloud Step 6 and a paragraph 76 from *Alcoholics Anonymous*.

After Step 5, I was already willing to ask God to remove my defects of character. I was clear that I was the maker of most of my misery and I truly wanted to be different.

It was at that moment that Kimmerz gave me a heads up that I'll never forget. "Oh, by the way," she said with a small smile, "just because you recognize these patterns of behavior doesn't mean you will be perfect from here on out. You are going to continue to make mistakes but it won't be nearly as often or as bad. You can clean it up by making amends."

Many of my relationships got better right away, as the pain of doing things the old way just wasn't worth it. One of the AA promises came true for me here, too: that I would intuitively know how to handle situations that previously baffled me. And when I didn't know what to do, Kimmerz gave me ideas on how to do things differently. She would say, "When in doubt, don't." Which meant that I didn't have to respond to people immediately and risk saying something I'd regret later.

They call this restraint of tongue and pen in the rooms. That idea has saved me from having to make amends more times than I can count. Sometimes I'd have to call her and run a situation by her to see how she would handle things. So many times I was like, "Wow, I never would have thought of that!" She said things like, "If you're still resentful at someone, pray for them that they should have all the things you want for yourself. Whatever you send out, comes back to you."

People are like mirrors. You can't love or hate something about someone else unless it's something you love or hate about yourself. If you spot it, you got it.

I remember hearing a spiritual teacher talk about having the courage to use this concept for self-awareness and transformation. It's not only a tool focused on transforming *negative* behavior patterns—it also works in the positive. If you love and admire someone, what you are seeing is the beauty and power that lies within you as well. In recovery, it is tempting to only focus on character defects but in order to maintain a balanced perspective and achieve emotional sobriety, we must consider the positives as well. What you focus on expands. So, yes, the moral inventory is important to identify what is not working and how to fix it—but then acknowledge your strengths and build on those, too.

Step 7: "Humbly asked him to remove our shortcomings."

Interpretation: When I feel myself repeating a negative pattern, I remember it is safe to ask the universe for help.

Principle: Humility

In this step, we will examine what humility is, why asking for help is significant, and how to identify what a shortcoming is. Step 7 is my favorite step. Mostly because whenever I find myself getting frustrated with relationships, or overly obsessed with an outcome, I come back to this step and review the ideas that help me to get "right sized."

When I met with Kimmerz to get my homework assignment for this step, she asked me to read Step 7 in *Twelve Steps and Twelve Traditions.* She suggested that every time I see the word "humility" I use a highlighter to drive home the point of how important it is, and the context in which it is used for deeper understanding of how I can apply it to my own life. Then, on a separate piece of paper, write down "Humility – the desire to seek and do God's Will" each time like a mantra to really let it sink in.

At first, this suggestion conjured up an image of Bart Simpson writing on a chalkboard as punishment. But in practice, it began the process of reshaping my subconscious beliefs about humility. My old ideas about humility were very negative and closely tied to humiliation. Feelings of shame, embarrassment, and disgrace. But as I soon learned, humility is very different.

When I am focused on humility—seeking and doing God's Will—I am in the process of getting quiet, of feeling grounded in the present moment, really going inside to listen for what feels right, so that I can take action and do the next right thing. I don't have to plan out my whole life in a fearful, controlling way. That's how I lived before getting sober, and it never worked out. Now I know I can live in the present moment and trust my heart enough to ask it for guidance.

Asking for help is built into this step for a reason. In the rooms you'll hear people talking about seeking "God's Will." When I first heard that sentiment, it was confusing to me. How are you supposed to know what constitutes your will and differentiate that from God's Will for all the different situations in your life? And how do you know your will or desires are not in alignment with God's?

I would suggest that as you practice self-care, and self-love, you will start to reconnect with your internal feelings better so they can guide your actions. The decisions and actions that bring you peace are closer to God's Will than having to manipulate, force, or control situations to get the outcome you want.

So why is it so hard to follow your own internal guidance?

I think there are a few reasons. For starters, most of us were not taught to trust our own feelings. As children we were told not to cry, or that we were being dramatic, or that we were ungrateful or selfish. These messages all say the same thing: Your feelings are not valid so don't trust them.

If we don't learn to acknowledge and honor our feelings, how can we develop the ability to tune into them? As a result, we learn to suppress our feelings and we become depressed and dysfunctional. We develop survival skills to compensate and distract us from our unprocessed pain. Some of these survival skills show up as addiction to substances, codependency, people pleasing, or needing external validation. That's why we must ask for help. We can get so locked into these survival skills that we feel stuck, and we need help to overcome them.

Much of recovery is spent unlearning things we learned as children. For instance, I was raised with religious ideas like "God won't do for you what you can do for yourself" which really speaks to the idea that we need to take action to fulfill our heart's desires, but that's not how I took it. I interpreted it to mean that God could help me, but he wasn't going to because I could do it all on my own.

When I was a little girl, I was often isolated when I was sad or angry to "work things out" on my own. It wasn't intentional, but the result was that I was repeatedly conditioned to isolate myself when I had negative feelings. Because I was not nurtured in those times of distress and taught how to process my feelings, I experienced benign neglect as a child. That type of conditioning reinforced my belief that I was alone and that I had to figure it out on my own.

So, it's no wonder that when I'm in distress as an adult it's not my natural instinct to seek help. It's something I must continually work at. There's a reason that "figure it out" is not a 12-Step slogan. It's because we need each other and a higher power to heal shortcomings. Kimmerz had me look up the definition of "shortcoming," which means "a fault or failure to meet a certain standard, typically in a person's character, a plan, or a system."

After doing Steps 4 and 5, I had new clarity on what my character flaws were. I kept hearing people at meetings talk so freely about their character defects, a term that still makes me bristle a bit. I prefer the term "human frailties." But hearing other people speak about their flaws so freely made it easier for my defenses to come down enough so I could get honest with myself. And as a result, I was relating to my new community more and more every day.

As I felt compassion for other members when they shared their experiences, I learned to have empathy and compassion for myself too. It was the first time I was able to see a balanced perspective when it came to how I saw myself.

When it comes to failing to meet a certain standard, these mostly showed up in my relationships. I learned that I needed God's help with some aspects of my character. I needed help in forgiving myself and others. I needed help managing my need to control people around me. I needed help taking responsibility for my actions and not being dependent on others for my own happiness. Mostly I learned that help was available, and with it, I could change.

Step 8: "Made a list of all persons we had harmed, and became willing to make amends to them all."

Interpretation: Starting with the people from my 4ᵗʰ step, I add all the people I hurt and ask for willingness to make amends to all of them.

Principle: Love

By this point in the process, I knew what was coming. I knew I was going to have to make amends to most of the people in my 4ᵗʰ step, as well as plenty of others I had no intention of speaking to ever again. There was no way I was going to speak to them, let alone bear my soul and apologize. Just the thought of talking to an ex-boyfriend, a former coworker, or a former friend was enough to make my heart race and my stomach churn with nausea.

Again, thank God for Kimmerz. She reminded me that all we had to do was make a list. That's it. That seriously took the pressure off. I could absolutely trick my mind into just making a list. The process of becoming willing to make amends to them ALL had to be done piecemeal in my case. After I made the list—with the easy ones at the top of course—I looked it over and thought, *How am I going to get to the place where I feel willing to tackle the rest?* Even though Kimmerz helped me see my part, it went against all my instincts to humble myself enough to reach out to some of those people and own my actions.

But I was missing the point. I wasn't going to make amends to them ONLY for their sake—I was doing it so I could be free of guilt and stay sober, too. This was also a practical opportunity to ask for help from my higher power.

In my heart, I honestly did not feel willing to make amends to a lot of those people. Kimmerz just asked me to keep praying for help, to pray for the people I felt the most resistance toward. She suggested something that sounded totally insane…to pray that they received all the forgiveness, happiness, peace, and joy I wanted for myself.

So that's what I did. All this time, I was still going to a lot of meetings, and it was strange how often the topic that day was exactly what I needed to hear. Also, enough time had passed that I was seeing some of the people I helped get sober relapse, which scared me to death. Since I was terrified of getting loaded again, it wasn't long before I just surrendered to the idea of simply owning my part so that I could stay sober.

Step 9: "Made direct amends to such people wherever possible, except when to do so would injure them or others."

Interpretation: Make amends to the people on my Step 8 list unless it would cause them, or others, additional harm.

Principle: Responsibility

I kept hearing that pain is the touchstone of all growth. I had gotten so uncomfortable sitting on my amends list that after I met with Kimmerz to go over it, I wanted to start knocking out the easy ones. But first she had me read Step 9 in *Alcoholics Anonymous* to make sure I was clear about my pattern of behavior, so that when I made amends I was able to acknowledge that pattern, how I hurt those involved, and then ask what I could do to make things right. Not just apologize.

Kimmerz and I had gone over my list thoroughly first. She'd said there was a reason we reviewed it together, mostly because it's not uncommon to want to make amends to people we really shouldn't, like an old drug dealer, or an ex that might still be using who could jeopardize my sobriety. She explained the difference between direct amends and living amends. Direct amends were to be made where it made sense, and living amends was a way of not continuing hurtful behavior—especially if I couldn't find the person on the list or if making amends would hurt them or others. There were two guys I dated that were married, so I knew I would not be meeting with them directly to make amends. My living amends would be to never behave that way in the future.

You know what surprised me the most about making amends? That some of the people I contacted didn't even remember the incidents I felt so bad about. I'd been carrying around so much guilt and shame over how I treated them! Most people forgave me instantly, and just told me to keep doing what I was doing. Like my parents. It was hard to make those amends. My heart was pounding as I told them it was important for me to take responsibility for my actions, and to share what I'd learned about myself. Maybe I'm lucky, but both of them said essentially the same thing—that they were just happy to have the real me back and that they were proud of me.

I worked through the list as fast as I could for fear of losing my nerve. After each one, I felt a little less guilty and a little more relieved. It was as if the burdens I'd been carrying around had been weighing me down, but once removed I felt as if I were floating. It's hard to describe the depth of my relief when I was done, but 30 years later I can still recall that feeling like it was yesterday.

Step 10: "Continued to take personal inventory and when we were wrong promptly admitted it."

Interpretation: By continuing to practice self-reflection, I can acknowledge positive character traits, while taking responsibility for mistakes, making amends when needed.

Principle: Discipline

Now that I was sober, had completed the moral inventory of all my resentments, recognized my patterns of behavior, and made amends where I could, I was moving into the last phase of the steps: how to maintain my sobriety.

Since life was still happening, I began to practice the 10th step on a daily basis as a way of establishing new habits. It helped me to manage my emotions and correct any mistakes I was making along the way. There was a lot to manage, considering I was working full time, in a relationship, and was developing many new friendships in the 12-Step rooms. So, Step 10 was a vital and ongoing process of self-examination to make sure I wasn't falling back into old behavioral patterns and staying on top of my resentments toward others.

Kimmerz and I were still meeting regularly. During this time, she asked me to keep a notebook next to my bed so that every night I could review my day by practicing the 10th step. I wrote down any new resentments, got in touch with what was being affected in me, and identified my part in the interaction. If I needed to make amends, I'd do it as soon as possible. It was a great learning process for me that gave me awareness to make different choices throughout the day. Especially because I hated making amends.

I have noticed my tendency is to think about problems I need to solve, but to stay balanced I also need to focus on what is working and celebrate the wins. I have learned that whatever we focus on expands, so it has been helpful to be less critical and practice more self-compassion. As part of the 10th step exercise, I listed things I had done well that day too such as moments when I practiced restraint, paused to consider God's Will, reached out to ask for help, or offered support. I listed all the self-care activities I did and acknowledged little moments of courage. It's a practice I have incorporated into my recovery that has really improved my self-esteem.

This practice has helped me to realize the promises as outlined in *Alcoholics Anonymous.*

The promises meant the world to me, even from the very beginning. They were often read at the meetings I attended regularly, and I trusted them wholeheartedly. They felt like a guarantee that if I did the work, I would experience the results for myself. In fact, over time these things did come true for me. Sure, the fear of financial insecurity and trusting in my higher power have tested me over the years but I found that when I returned to the steps I could find peace again quickly. That's one of the many benefits of going to meetings on a regular basis—I'm constantly exposed to ideas that keep me motivated to stay on the path.

Step 11: "Sought through prayer and meditation to improve our conscious contact with God as we understood Him, praying only for knowledge of His will for us and the power to carry that out."

Interpretation: As I practice prayer and meditation, the connection with my higher power grows, allowing me to follow my inner compass and tap into the power that is available to me.

Principle: Awareness

Throughout all the steps, Kimmerz had shared her experience with prayer and meditation. She'd already asked me to pray with her many times. Once we prayed in public, which was super embarrassing. I would rather be naked in public than pray in public, but I did whatever she asked me to in those days. We also prayed together when I did my 3rd step. It was a truly holy and intimate experience, one that changed me.

She said that prayer was talking to God, and meditation was listening. Praying on my own came easy to me, since I grew up in the Christian church. Kimmerz said it would strengthen my conscious contact with my higher power, and she was right. I used the prayers from *Alcoholics Anonymous*, and I said my own, too. Every morning I asked God for help to stay sober, and I recited prayers of gratitude at night. I'd heard in meetings that the one prayer that never failed was, "Thy Will be done," so I used that one a lot. I asked God for clear messages so I wouldn't miss them, and to be relieved of the pain caused by my own character defects. Throughout my life, I had given my power away by making other people responsible for my happiness, but now I wanted to reclaim my power by taking full responsibility for my actions and feelings.

By this time, I had been going to a few meditation groups to learn how to meditate. It was a lot different than I expected. I thought the goal was to clear my mind of all thoughts, and to achieve a state of Zen. In fact, that was pretty much the opposite of the instructions I got. In meditation, there are no goals, nothing to achieve, and nothing to do. The teachers would instruct me to sit comfortably with my back straight and hands on my lap, to settle into the present moment, and focus my attention on my breath. They told me to simply notice when I was lost in thought and bring my attention back to the breath. It was like fly fishing: I cast out my attention, and when I got lost in thought, I reeled it back to the present moment with no judgment, and no stress. They call it a practice for a reason.

Practicing in groups with a few people, or even in a big group at an ashram, were entirely different experiences from meditating alone. I loved meditating in groups because the energy was totally different. In groups, there were often candles, music, and incense. The noises from people shifting in their seats or coughing acted as reminders to return to the present moment. The energy felt more significant in some ways, more intense. When I practiced meditation on my own, I noticed I was able to quiet my mind better if I had done some physical exercise and journaling first. Exercise tired my body while journaling helped me process my feelings. A regular practice has become a vital part of my long-term recovery.

What I notice after a period of regular practice is that I feel noticeably calmer. It has been the antidote to my chronic anxiety. I seem to have the ability to pause before I react and make good choices in the moment. And It's not just me. If you do a quick internet search on meditation, you'll find countless scientific peer-reviewed journal papers on the benefits of meditation such as stress reduction, improved sleep, increasing brain cognition, and emotion regulation.

Step 12: "Having had a spiritual awakening as the result of these steps, we tried to carry this message to alcoholics, and to practice these principles in all our affairs."

Interpretation: I share my recovery experiences with others and continue to practice the principles of the program in all areas of my life.

Principle: Service

After completing the steps up to this point, my conscious contact felt stronger than ever before. It felt like everything was falling into place and I was able to respond to the natural rhythm of life. I was in a healthy relationship with another sober member, and I felt like I was in a good place. Of course there was still a lot I needed to learn, but I got comfortable with knowing I'd make mistakes but that I could stay sober with the help of my support system and my higher power.

Most of my direct amends had been made, I was relatively consistent with my morning self-care practice, and I was absolutely on fire for my sobriety. Personal growth was my favorite thing to talk about. My life was completely unrecognizable from the year before.

For Step 12, Kimmerz and I read Step 12 from the 12x12 together and Chapter 7 from the Big Book. Kimmerz said it was time for me to sponsor another woman and take her through the steps.

I was willing to do as she asked, but first I had to find someone who wanted a sponsor. I went to newcomer meetings and gave my phone number to as many women as I could. New members have a difficult time calling someone they barely know, so I eventually learned to get their number too and make the first call.

I'll be honest. In the beginning, I wasn't very good at it. In fact, I was totally confused as to what my role was. Somewhere along the line I began thinking it was my responsibility to "save" these women, and I was pretty controlling about it. I would get emotionally emmeshed, and often found myself getting entangled in other people's situations. I did everything wrong. I gave advice, I was overly protective, and I would even get upset over things that had nothing to do with me. But I learned from every experience.

Kimmerz helped me to see that my only job was to take women through the steps the way she had for me. I was not to give advice, but I could be honest about what came up for me as I listened. I could share my experience of what I would do if I were in that situation. She taught me to let go of any outcomes. People need to do what they feel is right and learn the lessons they need to learn. My role was to simply listen, redirect them to the step they were on, and to their higher power. She taught me that humility was knowing my limitations. To understand that, ultimately, I don't really know what's right for anyone else—and that I am not responsible for anyone else's decisions. I could offer positive encouragement and compassion and that was enough.

Over time, I developed better boundaries for myself and the women I worked with. To this day, if someone asks me to sponsor them I share how I do it, I ask them to sleep on it, and if they are ready to do whatever it takes to the best of their ability, only then do I agree. I ask that they do 90 meetings in 90 days, just as I did. I assign homework and when they have completed it, we schedule a meeting so they can share their work with me. I ask that they attend the same meeting I do at least once per week, so we can spend time together and I can introduce them to others who will become part of their support system. I ask them to get phone numbers of other members and to make at least 3 "willingness calls" per week—a call that demonstrates you are willing to take actions that support your sobriety, which include building a support system. There is no way I can be 100% available all the time, and when life happens, they need to be current with other members so that if I'm not available they have other people they can lean on. I have learned the hard way that if we don't call when we feel good, we have a very hard time calling when we feel like drinking.

Through mentoring others, I have also come to recognize my own personal limits. For instance, when we meet to go over homework I know I'm good for about an hour. After that my ADHD kicks in and I have a hard time focusing. Also, because of the work I do, I talk on the phone a lot. So, if someone calls and leaves a message, I may not call back right away unless I know it's urgent. I've asked the women I work with to use the pain scale, and to text me if they are at a 7 or above. Even if I'm in a meeting at work, I will get away as soon as possible to call them back. If it's not urgent and is simply a check-in call, I might call back the next day. If they are okay with all of that, we get into action.

Taking on a sponsorship role is such an honor. The fact that someone else sees something in me that they want, and that they trust me enough to share how they feel is a humbling experience. It makes me want to be the best version of myself that I can be.

They might not realize it, but they are helping me stay sober, too. I always make sure to explain that fact right away because when I ask them to call me as often as they need to, they all say they don't want to be a burden. It breaks my heart but I totally get it. I didn't want to be a burden to Kimmerz either but she gently insisted on it, which I am grateful for.

Being a sponsor has been so good for my sobriety. It keeps me focused on the solution, it allows me to be in service which builds my self-esteem, and it allows me to practice compassion for others. As a result, it helps me practice compassion for myself. I have come to understand that we can't escape the same measuring stick we judge others by. As I offer compassion to others, I learn to release the judgment I had for the things I have done. I learned that I am uniquely qualified to be useful to the women I sponsor because I understand how they feel. I get to share all the experiences I was ashamed of so that they don't have to feel alone in their experiences. It's such an intimate moment of connection to share empathy and have it received. Those are the moments when it feels like God is present and it's a high like no other.

Over the years, most of the women I sponsored either moved on to other sponsors, moved away, or left the program—but some have stuck with me for years. I have learned not to take it personally one way or the other. In fact, it's probably good to go through the steps with different people because everyone has something unique to offer.

If someone I sponsored relapsed, I used to feel personally responsible as if I had somehow failed them. It was a hard lesson, but now I understand I can't keep anyone else sober. If someone isn't ready to be sober, or if they need to learn something, there's nothing I can do or say to make them stay sober.

Over the years I have witnessed a variety of outcomes. I've seen people show up, do the work, and achieve long-term sobriety. I've seen people get long-term sobriety after years of relapsing as well. I've even known people who drink again and go on to live lives with the same ups and downs that I've had sober. I have been to a lot of funerals too. Not everyone survives this thing. It's heartbreaking and infuriating at the same time. I don't pretend to know why some people get it and others don't. At the end of the day, I feel so grateful that I've had the experience of living a sober life.

Nowadays, the message I try to impart—whether as a sponsor or when speaking at a meeting—is one of empathy, compassion, and hope. I consider it a great honor to be asked to share my story at a meeting. If someone asks me to sponsor them, I think about how much courage it took me to ask Kimmerz to be my sponsor, knees trembling and voice shaking.

And I'll always remember what she said, "It would be my honor. We'll start with Step 1."

7

Imperfectly Happily Ever After

How have the 12 steps affected my life since I quit drinking almost 30 years ago? I'm glad you asked. Let's get into it…

This section is broken down into the main areas of my life. The focus is on how the steps influenced my attitude, decision-making process, the actions I took, and the outcomes.

To be honest, my experiences since I quit drinking have been equal parts magical and hard. The magical part is that I have broken many negative behavior patterns since the beginning. Patterns I thought would never change. I'm no longer afraid to feel my feelings. I have learned how to process negative emotions to resolution and cultivate good feelings too.

The hard parts have been dealing with life on life's terms. It has been hard to feel grief when I've experienced loss like when someone I loved died. It has required a great deal of courage to heal from childhood trauma, or deal with a loved one's depression and addiction. But through this work, I have stayed sober through it all.

My Romantic Life

Bobby and I were very young when we met. I was newly sober at 25 and he was 24. He had already been sober for almost 6 years and had some practice managing his emotions. I did not. There was one instance where we got into an argument over something dumb and I lost my temper. I was pretty spicy then. My M.O. was to break shit and leave. I can still visualize a specific incident now.

We were standing in the living room of our apartment, and I was about to smash the shit out of his video game console. He stood in the way and was like, "Whoa! What are you doing?!" I must have sworn like a sailor and attempted to leave when he moved around to stand in front of the door. "Where are you going? We need to talk about this!" Keep in mind he's 6'1 and I'm 5'3. I wasn't going to be able to push him out of the way. We ended up sitting on the couch in uncomfortable silence. He would ask me, "Do you feel better?" I would say no, and he would say, "Then let's keep talking until we do."

Nobody ever did that for me before. He gave me a safe space to have my feelings, we had ground rules for tough conversations like no name calling or leaving (or in my case, no breaking things). We also agreed to keep talking until we both felt at peace.

In most cases where there was a disagreement we couldn't solve right away, we would take the issue to our sponsors and do a 4th step on it.

For instance, one night we went out to dinner with Ed and Leslie, my best friend and her boyfriend who had his own business and a lot of money. Ed wanted to leave a big tip and Bob agreed. I had huge triggers around money, and we were planning a wedding. We were struggling financially back in those days, and I felt like we needed to save as much as we could. I was so angry that Bob was willing to blow extra money just so he didn't have to look bad in front of Ed. I don't recall what I said, but I made it known that I was not happy and made everyone at the table uncomfortable. It was so awkward that Leslie suggested I go to the bathroom with her just to break the tension.

Later that night when I was able to call my sponsor, Julie, I unloaded the whole story on her. It was all about Bobby and how horrible he was with money, how he didn't give a shit about the wedding or how I felt. She listened until I ran out of steam and finally paused so she could respond. She asked me in a gentle voice, "Did you just want to vent, or do you want feedback? How can I support you right now?" I was floored.

Nobody had ever asked me that before. I asked for feedback, and she said, "Well, I don't sponsor Bobby, so let's look at your part." Again, I was floored, but this time I was pissed. I wanted her to take MY side. I was the victim in this scenario, right? Wrong! As we went through my resentments and got to my part, I was able to see how my behavior affected him, and frankly everyone at the table. Julie and I talked about what I could have done differently. We talked until I got to a place of empathy for Bobby for how I made him feel. Looking back, it's astonishing to realize how important it was for me to get to that place with Julie's help. She even provided me with compassionate support, so I didn't go into a shame spiral about my behavior when I was fearful and angry.

I was able to then go to Bobby, ready to own my part in that situation and let go of his part, which I had no control over. The beauty of this was since he's also practicing these principles, he went to his sponsor with this issue and they did the same thing. When Bobby and I came back together we were both focused on taking responsibility for ourselves and making amends to each other.

After 30 years together, this is still the process we use to resolve problems that arise, although with that much practice we have worked out nearly all our issues and rarely have arguments.

Parenting

There is a lot of marketing and mainstream messaging encouraging women to drink as a coping skill to parenting. It even has a name! It's called "mommy wine culture." I was fortunate that I had already been sober for eight years when I became a mother, and all my friends with children were sober too.

That doesn't mean parenting was easier but it did mean I had a support system, a regular self-care practice, and a practical process for stress management.

When the kids were little and I found myself being the primary caregiver, I became very resentful toward my husband. I felt responsible for carrying the load of all their physical and emotional needs and made all the childcare decisions. I was exhausted and full of self-pity.

Because I had a support system of other mothers who were sober and familiar with the 12-Step process, I had women who could easily spot errors in my thinking and offer practical solutions.

For instance, I was resentful that my husband never put the kids down for bed and it was a long and exhausting routine. So, I did a 10th step around it. I found that once I was able to name the exact cause of my resentment, "he didn't put the kids to bed," I could then name how it affected me. It affected my personal relationship with him and my self-esteem. I identified the fears: he didn't value my time, my mental health, I wasn't a good enough mother. Then I examined my part.

As it turned out, I was blaming him for not taking responsibility when I wouldn't LET him help me. It was MY belief that he had to do it MY way to be done the right way. I began to see how I had no boundaries with myself. I was totally selfish in thinking my way was the only way. As I went deeper, I realized I didn't value my own time, or my own mental health. I was the one that didn't believe I was worthy of rest or receiving help. I also realized I was holding him responsible for my feelings.

Once I started taking responsibility for my own feelings, setting boundaries for myself, asking for help when I needed it, and letting go of how things got done, the dynamics of our parenting partnership changed dramatically.

So instead of falling for the "mommy wine culture" way of dealing with stress, which is to numb it and check out, I was able to find the support I needed and identified specifically how I could change my behavior so I reduced my stress and resolved the resentment building up in my marriage. As a result, we have maintained a close, loving relationship through many parenting challenges.

Being sober also had a huge impact on how I relate to my children. I learned that if I was stressed out, it affected them too and they'd act out—reflecting back to me my own internal state. I learned that I had a tendency to deny my own need for rest, nourishment, and emotional support by putting everyone else's needs before my own. When I noticed this pattern, I was able to recognize that I was not being the kind of mother I wanted to be. I needed to make my own self-care a priority.

It changed how I set boundaries with the kids too. I used to ask them, "Do you want nice mommy, or mean mommy?" With wide eyes, they'd say, "We want nice mommy" because they knew that bitch was inches away from joining the party.

That story also reminds me that I learned to say I was sorry and make amends to my kids when I had made a mistake or hurt their feelings. I would let them know I was aware how my behavior hurt them. I would also give them a chance to tell me how they felt by asking them if there was anything they needed me to know. That wasn't something I had ever experienced growing up. I knew it was important to demonstrate to them that we all make mistakes, and how we take responsibility for our actions.

Relationships with Friends

My life prior to getting sober was filled with challenging friendships. I felt like I was good at making friends but not at keeping them. Growing up I would have one best friend who was typically very codependent. When I became an adult, my friendships were typically superficial or toxic. They didn't last very long so I would jump from friend to friend.

I used to feel so deeply sad and frustrated by the lack of friends I had in my life. I was terribly lonely and lost. Now it's obvious to me that I was the common denominator in all these relationships. But why was I like that? The answer was revealed through working the steps with a sponsor.

My sponsors would have me do a 10th step when I ran into conflicts with friends. For instance, Julie had me do one with a friend who didn't show up for my birthday dinner, we'll call her Samantha.

Here's how I wrote out the 10th step:

Resentful at: Samantha

The Cause: She didn't show up for my birthday dinner.

Affects My: Self-esteem, personal relationship, and emotional security.

Fear: She doesn't really care about me. I look bad because not enough people showed up to my party.

My Part: I had unreasonable expectations of her. I didn't appreciate the people who did show up. I had a belief that she needed to show up to be considered a good friend. I was selfish in depending on her for my happiness. I put conditions on our friendship. I gave my power away. I robbed myself of receiving joy at the party because I was focused on who didn't show up. I held a limiting belief about myself that I was nothing if everyone didn't show up for me. I didn't take her feelings or needs into consideration. I placed a huge burden on her to make me happy on my birthday, and when she couldn't meet that expectation, I withdrew my love for her. I was cold, angry, and I told her she wasn't a good friend. I was cruel and hurtful to her. I talked mad shit behind her back to our mutual friends.

The last section where I examined my part didn't come easily to me. That's always where I have needed the most help. For that I have always chosen sponsors who have been direct and honest, yet gentle and compassionate because facing the truth about my behavior was often shame-provoking for me.

I was lucky to have women in my life who would remind me not to be too hard on myself. They would explain that since I was carrying around abandonment trauma, low self-esteem, and had never been taught healthy coping skills, it was inevitable I would react this way when I felt hurt. Now having a broader understanding of what was really going on inside me, I had clarity and could take steps to rectify the situation.

Once I am clear on my part, and reach a place of empathy for how my behavior has affected others, I can take responsibility, ask for suggestions on what to do instead, and change my behavior.

Today I have a wealth of friends and what used to confuse me in friendships now is second nature to me.

Work and Career

When I look back over my career since I got sober, I can't imagine the decisions I would have made had I not had the practice of applying the 12-Step principles in my life.

One of the most challenging and painful experiences I had early on in sobriety was working for a large high-tech company in Silicon Valley, California. A new position had been created in the HR department to handle the new hire process which also included mergers and acquisitions and the student intern program. Because it was a newly created position, all they had was an estimation of the workload. In practice, it was an extremely complicated role that underestimated the amount of time required to complete all the tasks. I was over-whelmed and completely stressed out. My manager and I would have regular meetings where I would ask for more help and he would tell me I needed to work more efficiently.

It got so bad that they put me on a process improvement plan which was a huge source of shame for me. I had never worked so hard while feeling so underappreciated and misunderstood. It was an incredibly painful time for me, but I was able to stay sober by applying the principles of the program.

Every time I had resentment toward my manager, or a coworker, I would talk it out with my sponsor first to process my feelings. Then, I would pray and ask for guidance, followed by a 10th step writing exercise. Although it was a very challenging time in my life, I learned a lot about myself. That was probably one of the first times I had a practical example of how my self-esteem was directly tied to external approval. My boss was not involved in the day-to-day activities, so he was relying on my coworkers to report back. I was under a ton of stress because of the workload and deadlines I was managing. My coworkers often worked with me to get everything done on time. Unfortunately, we didn't have the same work styles, so we were often in conflict. Because I was ultimately held responsible if something didn't get done on time, I would be the one driving the process. I didn't know how to handle the stress or communicate my needs very well.

Looking back, I can see that my need for my manager's approval was so strong I would get angry with my coworkers and say things I would later regret. Since my boss was relying on them for feedback, and because I was so angry, they would give him negative reports about my performance and tell him the workload was reasonable.

By writing out the 10th step and reviewing it with my sponsor, I was able to deconstruct the situation, identify my thought and behavior patterns, and take responsibility for my actions. I made amends to my coworkers for my part and continued to do my best until I was able to find another job that I was better able to manage.

It was an incredibly humbling experience, but it brought to light many lessons I needed to learn about the root causes of how I think and what I believe. I learned to manage my feelings with prayer and meditation so I didn't give into saying hurtful things. I learned how to improve my self-esteem by doing acts of service to find peace within myself. I also learned how to let go of other people's perceptions of me and focus on being more empathetic to myself.

Things have a funny way of working out in ways I could not have predicted. As it turned out, the person who replaced me went out on stress leave a month after assuming the role, and they had to hire three people to do the job I was doing alone. That showed me that my value was always there, even if the people I was working with didn't see it.

This practice of applying the 12-Step principles to my work life led me to an amazing career as an Account Executive working for Fortune 100 companies and exciting tech startups in Silicon Valley. There were many challenges to say the least.

Every time I was facing something that felt overwhelming, I would go to my 6am meeting to get grounded before work. Just walking into the room, I would feel my shoulders drop and I would take a deep breath. The sense of belonging, love, and connection would bolster me for the day. Honestly, I don't know how other people cope without having something like this. It's no wonder that there is a mental health crisis.

Spirituality

Before I got sober, I had completely abandoned all forms of spirituality. The program offered me a new way to think about spirituality that is separate from religion. Having that perspective allowed me to be more open to spirituality and gave me practices like prayer and meditation that added new depth and meaning to my life. It also gave me a way to connect with my internal guidance and with other people.

Because I attended meetings regularly, I heard so many stories of how having a new concept of a higher power and a spiritual practice helped others stay sober. Their stories of serendipity would get past the walls of my heart and open my skeptical mind. The stories I heard had a profound effect on me and it helped me to cultivate my own experiences of feeling guided, supported, and open to new possibilities.

Maryann was one of my early sponsors, and one day she walked into a meeting I was speaking at. While telling my story, I happened to mention my exact sobriety date, which I normally don't do. When I finished, I chose a topic and began to call on people to share as was the custom in that meeting. When I called on Maryann, she said she would like to pass her time to a woman I had never seen before. I don't recall her name, but I'll never forget what happened.

This woman shared that her husband had just died and that she was on her way to his service after the meeting. She was understandably grief-stricken. She said she didn't want to drink so decided to go to a meeting first. Then as she shared how sad, scared, and alone she had felt, she said she couldn't believe it: when I shared my sobriety date, it felt like a message from God. As it turned out, my sobriety date was their wedding date! The room fell silent. Something shifted and we all felt it. It was like we all felt connected to something greater than ourselves. She said it felt like a sign that he was still with her and that everything was going to be okay. She felt a sense of relief and peace that would carry her through her beloved's service.

Everyone that shared after commented on how powerful the experience was. It was truly undeniable.

That's what having a spiritual practice feels like. It's experiences like that that have happened many times in my sobriety, yet I'm always amazed. After all the experiences I've had, my default is to forget that I'm not alone and I don't need to figure things out. But that's why they call it a practice. Some days are better than others and I will always have to work against my skeptical mind. That is why I continue to practice connecting with a higher power through prayer and meditation.

Creating a New Identity

About 20 years into my sobriety, I shared my story at a woman's recovery facility. Driving up the long and windy road in my little 325 BMW, after a day of working at a prestigious tech company in professional dress and heels, I was feeling a bit anxious about how I would be received. After all, I had never been to a treatment center and I just didn't know if they would relate to me.

My fears increased when I walked in. Most of the women there came straight from jail or as an alternative to jail. There were lots of tattoos; shabby, ill-fitting clothes; wildly unkempt hair; missing teeth; and many had scabs on their faces that were still healing from "tweaker face" as they called it.

Just based on appearances, I was worried they weren't going to want to hear my story based on how I looked. The truth is, I was judging them based on how *they* looked.

As they gathered and sat in their seats, and quieted down, the meeting organizer began to read from the 12-Step literature and a sense of calm washed over me. I was reminded of my purpose; to carry the message of hope to those who are still suffering.

I began to share my story of what it was like. The feelings of never quite fitting in or belonging anywhere, not even in my own family. Feelings of self-loathing as I drank uncontrollably and behaved in ways I was deeply ashamed of. I shared the feelings of loneliness and the hopelessness I felt that nothing would ever be different. As I continued to share from my heart, the room became still and quiet. I could see in their eyes that they understood me. Pain recognizes pain.

I felt so connected to them in those moments. So grateful for the space they gave me to share and unburden myself. I got to tell them about all the amazing women who had supported me along the way, and how that kind of love allowed me to forgive myself and even love myself. I shared how through a lot of hard work, I became a good mother, a cherished wife, a considerate friend, a loving daughter, a caring sister, and a dependable employee.

In that moment I realized I had become a version of myself I could be proud of. I was able to share from my heart and offer hope—yet in return, I was able to receive love and acceptance for who I am.

Finances

Financial insecurity has always been something I have wrestled with. Growing up, the lack of money was always an issue. To be clear, my parents were both honest, decent, hardworking people. However, they divorced when I was about seven and some of my earliest memories include hearing my parents talk about how there was never enough of it. My dad would express stress and frustration about how much he had to pay in child support or deny our requests to go do fun things because everything was too expensive.

My mother was always going to extremes to save money too, like never turning on the heater and telling us to put on a sweater instead. Fortunately, we lived in California so it's not like it snowed, but the thermostat was definitely not something we were ever allowed to touch. We never threw food away either. I remember my mom coming home from a date and she brought home the heel of the bread and individually wrapped squares of butter in a little bag. I was so embarrassed for her!

The worst times were when she was working as a teacher's aide and she only got paid once a month. At the end of the month our cupboards would be bare as we waited for the next paycheck. We had two dogs that suffered the most because if we ran out of dog food, they had to wait. My sister and I would try to feed them anything we could find. Like maybe a random can of soup, or old dry cereal. I'll never forget the guilt and powerlessness I felt because I knew they were starving and there was nothing I could do about it.

These painful experiences of lack turned into negative beliefs that were deep-seated in my subconscious. Beliefs that there was never enough money, that I had to work hard and struggle to get money, and that I was powerless to respond to unexpected events that caused me to lose money. My underlying beliefs about money were tied to pain, suffering, and powerlessness. They were also tied to my self-worth. Since there wasn't enough money when I was growing up, my needs or desires were often secondary to what my parents deemed to be the priority. I often didn't have appropriate clothes and felt the shame of not fitting in at school. Although I made the drill team in high school I was forced to quit when my dad found out how much it cost, which was devastating to my self-worth.

After I got sober, I still had significant fears about money that kept showing up as an adult. My husband and I could barely talk about money without it turning into a huge fight. He complained that I was stingy and controlling and I felt he was frivolous and irresponsible.

What helped me more than anything else was doing the 10th step on a regular basis. It was a very pragmatic and practical way for me to focus on what I could control and let go of what wasn't within my control. It also helped me to identify all the fears that were driving my feelings and behavioral patterns.

By having this conscious awareness, I could find ways to mitigate my fears and choose to adopt a healthier mindset and take more productive actions. I leaned heavily on my support system for this. I belonged to a huge fellowship and had access to tons of people who were better at relationships and money issues than I was. I also leaned heavily on my concept of a higher power for guidance, peace, and to put the right people in my path.

We have had many challenges around money over the years and I have always come back to using the principles I learned in the program. Today I have financial freedom and the fear of economic insecurity has left me.

Family Relationships

When I first got sober, my relationships with my family were in rough shape. Considering that after years of taking them for granted, and behaving selfishly, they were surprisingly tolerant of me—especially my dad and stepmom. They had repeatedly helped me financially when I prioritized spending money on weed and alcohol instead of paying rent or my car payments.

My mom would never help me that way, but at the end of my drinking I had been living with my boyfriend and when we broke up, she let me move back in with her and my sister. She had been renting out my old room, so she gave a 30-day notice to her tenant so that I could have it back. Meanwhile, I slept on her couch. I think she let me move back in because she could see I was in bad shape. I had been very depressed and couldn't eat much. I was just under 100lbs and I think she was scared for me.

Those first 90 days of being sober were tough, but they were also magical in a lot of ways. My mom kept saying, "It's so good to have the real Arlina back." She was right. I was increasingly becoming myself as I started taking care of myself again. My sister and I had never been closer. She was going with me to 12-Step meetings all the time and gave me so much support.

Over the years my relationships with my parents got so much better. I began to accept them for who they were, limitations and all. Although I realized there were some things I couldn't share with my mom such as my emotional pain. She simply couldn't be supportive in the way I needed her to be. If I tried to process my feelings with her, she would either skip over them or minimize them. If it had to do with my childhood or how the divorce affected me, she would say things like, "I don't regret it. It was the best thing for me." Totally dismissing the profoundly negative impact it had on me. Not that I think they should have stayed married, but there was no validation of how hard it was for me and my sister.

I learned not to take my pain to her. With the help of my support system, I was able to have some compassion for how she grew up and learned to cope with negative feelings. I began to appreciate the absolutely incredible woman that she was. She was by far the most positive person I have ever met, with this uniquely effervescent and sparkly personality that everyone loved. I consider myself so fortunate that she was my mom. And when she was diagnosed with terminal cancer, I got to be the one who slept beside her bed for the remainder of the 22 days she was alive. I got to hear her say goodbye to all her friends who loved her so much and thanked her for all the times they shared together, the good and the bad. These are among the most precious moments of my life.

Unfortunately, not all my family relationships endured. Although my sister and I had been close while I was getting sober, I met Bobby early on and didn't spend much time with her anymore.

As I worked through the steps, I attempted to make amends with her a few times, but our relationship was never close again. In fact, it continued to get worse. What I have come to accept is that it takes two people to do the work and if one person isn't willing to participate, sometimes it's better for both to let go with love. It has taken me decades to finally find a place of peace and acceptance around that relationship. There is still sadness that things aren't different, but I know in my heart that my responsibility is to protect my peace.

I still consider myself extremely blessed to have such a good relationship with my stepbrother and stepmother. They are truly the most compassionate, loving, and caring people you'd ever be fortunate enough to meet. I think back to when my stepmother sat with me and gave me a safe place to live when I could no longer live with my mom when I was 14 years old. I'm sure it was hard on her to have such an angry, dysfunctional girl in her home, but she always treated me with such compassion and endless patience. She was a saint. I'll be eternally grateful to her for giving me the nurturing I longed for but never got from my own mom.

My stepbrother and I had always been close and continue to be to this day. He is a treasure to me and has always been there to support me through all of life's challenges. I consider myself blessed to have him in my life.

Healing and Personal Growth

Getting sober was just the beginning of my healing process. The 12-Step program was foundational in many ways because it provided critical elements I needed for a healthy life. Like community, connection, service, and a regular review of the solutions that kept me on a path of healing and personal growth.

The community aspect was vital to my mental health in that I had a place to go and meet people on the same path, working toward the same goal. While it gave me a place to share my feelings and have them validated, the groups I had access to were solution-oriented. The way people shared was largely from experience, not hyperbole. They talked about challenges they had and the actions they took to overcome them. Repeatedly, I would hear people say things like, "I don't know what's right for you, but here's what I did when I was in that situation." I was encouraged to "run the experiment" for myself. It was less about giving advice and more about offering suggestions. People who had what I wanted had more credibility than those who didn't, so it shaped who I went to for support or feedback.

By taking actions that were recommended, I began to see results. I learned to love the discomfort of self-examination because I knew it would lead to relief in the end. It is a practice that has served me over three decades to overcome long-standing behavior patterns.

There have been times when I took less action that contributed to my mental health, and I would go back to familiar ways of coping and negative thought patterns. What got me back on track is my connection with the people in my community and having a spiritual practice that provides comfort, direction, and a sense of purpose that is greater than myself.

While I have come to accept that there will always be a need to continue to practice self-care to maintain my mental health, I no longer believe I am broken. I do believe that a peaceful, joyful, purposeful life is available to me—and anyone who seeks it—one day at a time.

PART 2

The Foundation

8

The Lowdown on Booze Addiction: What it is and What it's Not

Before we go any further, it's helpful to understand the science behind alcohol and how it effects our body and psychology. When we look at addiction from a medical standpoint, this allows us to separate the emotion surrounding addiction from the science. It becomes clear that alcohol addiction is not a shameful moral failing. Instead, addiction is the inevitable conclusion for those of us that regularly consumed alcohol. This realization allowed me to have more compassion for myself, in turn helping me to accept the ideas, solutions, and practices that helped me heal from alcohol addiction.

Let's start with the neuroscience behind alcohol addiction. Alcohol causes your brain to release dopamine and endorphins that creates a pleasurable feeling and can initially reduce social anxiety. It is very easy to become dependent on alcohol to relieve anxiety and stress. However, alcohol raises your baseline of cortisol—the stress hormone—when you are not drinking, so alcohol becomes the cause of stress. It makes sense that at the end of a long day, you begin to feel the urge to have a drink to relax and it turns into a habit. Once it becomes a habit, it often turns into a mental obsession, becoming the focal point of your life. It becomes the center of every event, rather than an enhancement.

Also, alcohol is classified as a carcinogen associated with many terminal diseases such as cirrhosis of the liver; and many types of cancer including oral, pharynx, larynx, esophagus, colon, rectum, and breast. Alcohol is both water soluble and fat soluble, so it can penetrate and damage every cell of the body. By cutting alcohol out of your life, you could be saving your own life—and possibly the lives of others.

Even knowing how harmful drinking alcohol can be, quitting is not easy. There is a lot of external pressure to drink in just about every social situation. It's so easy to start planning activities around drinking that it is often the focus and over time it becomes addictive. There is a lot of resistance to the word "addiction" but in the simplest terms, addiction is quite simply the narrowing of things that bring you pleasure. Hobbies, friends, and loved ones become less and less important as the focus increasingly becomes alcohol.

Alcohol-use disorder, or alcoholism, is considered to be progressive. As an individual's drinking accelerates, their tolerance increases as well. More alcohol is required to produce the same effect, which perpetuates the drinking cycle.

Those who become physically addicted often need to medically detox. To stop drinking abruptly—with no medical supervision—could lead to severe symptoms of withdrawal, such as nausea, vomiting, hallucinations, seizures, and even death.

But the problem with using alcohol to regulate one's feelings isn't just physical. It may work to numb feelings temporarily but using alcohol only masks existing problems and creates new ones—thereby compounding stress, damaging relationships, and creating additional emotional pain. In other words, alcohol creates more problems than it solves.

9

The Battle With Recovery Resistance

Make no mistake, if you are going to start down the path of recovery, you will experience internal resistance. The resistance will arise when you hear ideas that challenge your current belief system. I know I'm bumping up against resistance when I get angry. So that's fun! I've come to accept when I get triggered like that, when I get really defensive, that's my signal that I need to dig a little deeper into my beliefs. To be fair, most people who want to get sober want to do it within their existing belief system, so you are not alone!

The way to get around that barrier is to realize that if you could get sober within your current belief system, wouldn't you have done it already? The truth is there is something within your belief system that is limiting your growth; we'll call that a limiting belief. Don't freak out, it's not your fault! The foundation of our beliefs about ourselves and the world are established by the time we are around eight years old, maybe even younger.

We have experiences, interpret those experiences, and conclude what they mean. We then look for reasons why our conclusions are correct, which entrenches that belief. That process is called confirmation bias. It's one of the biggest obstacles to growth so we must be open-minded enough to reconsider ideas that challenge our long-held beliefs about ourselves, other people, and how the world works.

Now might be a good time to ask yourself, *Would I let an eight-year-old make decisions about my life, what I should do, or who I am?* I would hope not! But if we don't take the time to deconstruct our beliefs that's exactly how we are operating in the world. When we are young, we lack context, experience, and perspective so it's natural that we develop inaccurate beliefs.

There are two main types of limiting beliefs; beliefs based on false information and/or missing information. As an example: When I was young I would run up to mom, shouting about something I was excited about, only to have her snap at me and yell at me for interrupting her. I would then feel hurt, interpret that experience as rejection, and conclude that I'm not good enough. Repeat that experience ad infinitum and I had a belief that I am "not lovable" which turned me into an achievement junkie. As an adult, it's the belief that drives my ambition, for better or worse.

This particular belief is based on both a false belief and missing information. It's objectively false because I know my mother did in fact love me. It's also missing information. What I didn't know at the time was that my mother was completely stressed out and overwhelmed. She wasn't entirely angry with *me*; she was just tired and had no reserve to draw from to practice patience in that moment. But as a child, I didn't know that and took her response to mean there was something wrong with me. This belief was then internalized subconsciously and deeply affected my self-esteem.

You might be wondering what all this has to do with recovery resistance. Well, here's how I think of it: Recovery resistance comes from the subconscious beliefs and feelings that keep us stuck in negative thoughts and behavior patterns. Resistance to new ideas and to taking different types of action based on fear and avoidance. It's the procrastination we experience when faced with taking action toward reaching our goals. At the core of recovery resistance is the confrontation of our established identity. Our identity that defines who we believe we are and how we relate to the world, and the coping strategies we develop to survive. I say it's who we *believe* we are because there is a difference between who we actually are and the persona we develop to survive in the world. We might think of ourselves as it relates to the roles we play, how we look, or what we have achieved.

When I think of my identity in those terms, I might say I'm a mother, wife, and friend. Or I would say I'm short, middle-aged, and fair-s'kinned. Or I would say I'm a writer, a teacher, and podcaster. However, those identifiers do not relate to my character traits. Traits like selfish or generous, honest or dishonest, lazy or hardworking, prideful or humble. Most of us land on the spectrum of these character traits to varying degrees. If we are to grow, an honest appraisal of where we are is required—but that's exactly what brings up resistance. It is incredibly difficult to identify where we might actually be lying to ourselves.

As they say, it's hard to read the label from inside the jar. Just like when a friend tells you about their relationship issues, you can quickly see a potential solution although they are seemingly blind to it. This is because they are reacting emotionally, and emotions often skew one's perceptions. You are not emotional about their situation which is why you can see things clearly when they can't. This is another reason why the program and meetings work so well together. It is a community of people who are on a similar journey, with similar issues, using similar terminology—all striving for the same goal of sobriety. We practice mindfulness through this process because unconscious limiting beliefs will keep you from seeing new opportunities and trap your mind in a loop of negativity. Keeping an open mind is essential for recovery.

So, it makes sense why we have recovery resistance, but what are some other ways we can identify it? The AA literature talks about how most of us try to hold onto our old ideas, but that we often can't quit for good until we let go of them. This tells me that if we are not getting the results we want, there are subconscious beliefs we need to deconstruct. For me, it was a process of trial and error before I had the ability to let go.

As we learn new ideas, we test it out against long-held beliefs or ideas. When we can accept that the old ideas aren't leading to the results we want, that's when we're able to let go of them. We literally surrender them.

First, here are examples of "old ideas" in the context of recovery from alcoholism:

Thinking we could:

Quit drinking without help
Moderate our drinking
Hang out with people who are drinking when we're just starting out
    in our sober journey
Ruminate on resentments
Drink only if something tragic happens or to celebrate an event

Other ideas include:

Not making recovery the number 1 priority
Thinking we need to control others to be happy
Letting go of our ideas about what relationships are supposed to be
The idea that our drinking behavior isn't selfish or self-centered
Thinking we need someone or something in our lives to be happy
The idea that we have to endure toxic people or environments
Thinking others were to blame for our feelings

The main cause of resistance are ideas that challenge existing beliefs and our identity, but procrastination and self-sabotage are also internal blocks that create recovery resistance.

Everyone struggles with procrastination on some level. If we all just did what we know to do, our lives would be heavenly. So why do we procrastinate? It's typically because the work of recovery is perceived as painful in some way. The work feels too big, too hard, it will take too long, or we don't have any evidence to believe the pain will ever be resolved. However, if we recognize that limiting beliefs are what's keeping us stuck, we can do some self-examination to identify the belief that is holding us back, ask other people in recovery for help, and start taking baby steps toward doing the work.

Here are some tips to help you overcome procrastination:

1. Recognize that this is a stress response. Take a moment to offer yourself some compassion. Doing something new is stressful, especially when it involves facing thoughts and feelings you have been avoiding.
2. Practice "chunking". Take the task at hand and break it down into tiny little steps.
3. Commit to taking action for two minutes at a time.
4. Do a three-second countdown and MOVE. Don't think, just move. Momentum will carry you the rest of the way.

Most people think they will take action when they feel motivated—but science has shown that motivation comes after taking action, not before. Mood follows action.

You might be wondering how to spot a limiting belief, so I would like to offer a simple writing exercise in lieu of an explanation. On a piece of paper, without judgment or self-editing, write down all the reasons why you haven't stopped drinking yet. Once you have listed everything you can think of, go back to the top of the list.

The reasons you list hold the clues to your limiting beliefs.

For instance, if you listed "I want to quit drinking, but I feel like I deserve a glass of wine at night to relax," the underlying limiting belief might be that you need alcohol to relax or that you can limit yourself to having just one drink. Most people don't really challenge their own thinking. A couple of good questions to ask yourself for each reason you listed is, "Is that really true?" or "What else could I do instead?". Something else to consider is asking other sober people how they handle the challenges you listed.

Now let's consider self-sabotage, which is a pattern of behaviors or thought patterns that prevents someone from achieving their goals and negatively impacts their well-being. In neuroscience terms, our brains have something called the default mode network, which is similar to the operating system in a computer. It is responsible for how the brain is wired, how it develops patterns of thinking, and in turn, how those affect our behavior. It creates a comfort zone of sorts and acts as a thermostat that keeps us from getting too high or too low.

When we enter recovery, we are actively doing the work to raise the thermostat to improve the quality of our lives, but this is when recovery resistance kicks in. We subconsciously self-sabotage our progress so that we can remain within our established comfort zone. Intellectually, we can think we want to make progress, but subconsciously we have a deep desire to stay safe. This desire comes from a primal belief that our old ideas have helped us to survive this long, so on a deep level, we resist actions that will take us to places outside our comfort zone, even if they are positive. The good news is this default is something that we can change through step work and therapy.

The steps are the application of principles for healthy living. It's the daily practice of those principles that over time becomes second nature and resets the default mode network. It's an ongoing practice because just as you wouldn't expect to eat one salad and stay healthy forever, or save one dollar and expect to retire, it is unreasonable to think that you can do the work of getting sober, then revert to past behaviors, and expect to stay sober. Without continuous practices such as self-examination, meditation, connection, service, and emotional management, our brain is wired to return to default mode.

Self-sabotaging behaviors can be conscious or unconscious and can manifest in many ways. Some examples of self-sabotaging behaviors include:

Choosing to drink again after a period of sobriety
Switching addictions
Picking a fight to excuse drinking
Failing to practice self-care
Forgetting important events or dates
Feeling unable to move forward in the face of a positive opportunity

Here are some ideas to overcome self-sabotaging behaviors:

1. When you make a mistake, let the pain burn you a little bit so the next time you feel tempted to sabotage, you remember how bad you felt. The next time you are tempted to make the same mistake, let the memory of the pain detour you.

2. Cultivate a sense of self-esteem, self-worth, and safety through service. If we don't believe we deserve to feel at peace, we will self-sabotage to stay in our dysfunctional comfort zone.

3. Seek out an Internal Family System (IFS) professional to help you resolve internal blocks so you can break through to the next level.

10

Rocking The Recovery Mindset

The recovery mindset is the attitude and thoughts you hold while learning about recovery. Approaching the 12-Step program with an open mindset will help you to get the most out of the process so you can quit drinking and lead a productive life. It's about having the humility to realize that what you have been doing isn't working, and being open to new ideas and taking suggestions—even if they don't seem to make sense at first.

To be fair, most people aren't usually super excited at the idea of joining AA. I know I wasn't. Concluding that I needed help was a painful and scary process all by itself. By the time I got to that place, I felt afraid, humiliated, and confused. I thought, *How did I end up here?* I was conflicted about going to AA because I dreaded the idea, but on the other hand I knew drinking was ruining my life and I hadn't been able to stop on my own. I was so tired of the struggle that I had reached the point of surrender. I was willing to try anything at that point, including AA.

My friend Mitch had already introduced me to the idea of H.O.W. The acronym that stands for Honesty, Open-Mindedness, and Willingness and since I was going to try this thing, I had an opportunity to put it into practice.

Think of honesty as the ability to recognize reality and see things as they truly are. It is a reliance on facts without emotion. No true progress can be made without an honest appraisal of the current situation.

There's a lot of talk about "cash register honesty". This obvious kind of honesty is if a cashier gives you too much change, you are honest enough to acknowledge what happened, open-minded enough to understand you'll feel good about yourself if you give it back and have a willingness to do so. It's the kind of thought process that is focused on behavior and making the right choice. That seemed easy enough for me to understand.

What was harder was all the subtle ways I was lying to myself. Like saying I was fine when I wasn't (At some point I heard the anacronym for FINE. Fucked up, insecure, neurotic, and emotional). Or telling myself I didn't care when someone hurt my feelings because I didn't have the courage or skill to speak my truth. Or hiding my self-centered motives behind good ones. Like venting about someone to a friend when really all I was doing was character assassination and trying to seek validation or make myself look better than them. Instead, I was learning to be willing to take responsibility for my feelings, find the courage to speak directly to the people I had a problem with, and open-minded enough to hear them out and consider how they felt.

After understanding how dishonest I had been with myself and others, it was tempting to take things to the other extreme and be too honest. I learned the hard way that honesty without compassion was cruelty. It didn't feel good to be cruel, so I learned to say what I mean, mean what I say, but to not say it mean. For me, honesty in relationships is a practice.

There was also the matter of practicing H.O.W. in my critical thinking skills. If I was going to put this idea into practice, I had to consider that my way of thinking wasn't working. As other people at meetings say, "My best thinking landed me in AA".

This is how my thinking played out: I had a belief about who I was, I made a decision based on that information, and then I took action. So, before I got sober, my belief was that I was a just a party girl. Someone who liked to have a good time and had a high tolerance for alcohol. I would often brag that I could drink men twice my size under the table.

My decision was to drink as much as I wanted because I believed I could. The problem with my thought process was that I was in denial of the outcome. The truth was I paid a heavy price in hangovers and shame for my drunken behavior. In fact, I could not drink as much as I wanted without impunity.

Open-mindedness allowed me to reconsider long-held beliefs in every area of my life and to seek additional information. This was the process of letting go of all my old ideas that were keeping me trapped in the cycle of suffering.

With a mindset of honesty, open mindedness, and willingness I learned there were errors in my belief system. I was able to see my own patterns clearly, gather new information, take different actions, and experience different—and better—results, in all areas of my life.

There is another way of looking at the recovery mindset. It's the growth mindset vs. the fixed mindset. Carol Dweck is an American psychologist at Stanford University, known for her research on motivation and mindset. She argues that there are two types of mindsets: a growth mindset and a fixed mindset.

People who have a growth mindset believe their intelligence and abilities can be developed with hard work, persistence, and practice. People with a fixed mindset do not. They typically blame others for how they feel and how their life has turned out.

People who go through the 12-Step program with a growth mindset demonstrate a willingness to face their challenges, are open to new ideas and feedback, and are able to see setbacks as learning opportunities. They are the ones you see at meetings who share their feelings and learning experiences while going through the steps. They are often the ones who lead meetings and do service work. They offer positive encouragement to others and are willing to seek guidance from people with more experience than they have.

People with a fixed mindset will spend a lot of time talking about the problem and do not take the suggestions offered to them. They keep doing things their way, blame others for how they feel, and wallow in self-pity. They are unwilling—or unable in some cases—to take the actions necessary for change. It's been my experience that people who start off with a fixed mindset can change and adopt the growth mindset. It helps to see the growth mindset in action. Going to meetings and watching others demonstrate the growth mindset is inspiring.

This is where sponsorship plays a role in moving someone from a fixed mindset to a growth mindset. It starts with something I call identity shaping. It's when you ask yourself, *What kind of person do I want to be?* List all the character traits of the people you admire most, then start working on embodying those character traits.

With that said, I ask that you try and lean into the discomfort of the growth mindset. I know it can be challenging, as it will require you to set aside thinking that no longer serves you in exchange for a new outlook. One that delivers both relief and freedom.

11

Why 12-Step Programs Are Awesome

There are many options for treatment available nowadays, so why should anyone even consider giving this program a shot? I could tell you that it is a well-tested program that has helped millions of people worldwide ever since it was founded in 1935, and that those who take suggestions, work the steps, and take consistent action usually succeed in time—even if they experience a period of relapses.

But that is boooorrrring...not to mention pedantic. And, quite honestly, you've probably heard it all before. So, let's get personal.

I was attracted to the program because I was isolated and terribly lonely. As I mentioned, I had ruined nearly all my friendships due to my drinking, and the program was full of people who were both welcoming and nice to me. They talked openly about things I was ashamed to say out loud, which immediately piqued my interest and kept me coming back. For the first time in my life, I felt like I belonged somewhere. I found the "younger" meetings, so I could make new friends close to my own age and have fun.

I heard powerful messages from others that touched my heart and gave me hope. As I went through the steps, I began to experience incredible insights, establish priceless friendships, and amassed many spiritual experiences—all of which kept me coming back. Overall, I felt better and had new hope for the future!

Another reason 12-Step programs are awesome is that it is widely accepted to be one of the most effective treatments available for little to no cost. There is much critical discussion about the success rate of the 12 steps. Some say that since there is no empirical data because it is an anonymous program, the effectiveness cannot be verified. However, several studies have shown the effectiveness of Alcoholics Anonymous (AA) and its 12-step approach in treating alcohol use disorder (AUD). A comprehensive review published by the Cochrane Library analyzed 35 high-quality studies involving over 10,000 participants and concluded that AA is more effective at achieving long-term abstinence compared to other interventions like cognitive behavioral therapy (CBT). The review highlighted that AA's benefits increase over time, with participants showing higher rates of abstinence at 12, 24, and 36 months compared to those receiving professional therapy alone.

One reason for AA's success is its peer-led, socially supportive environment, which fosters a sense of belonging and accountability. Participants in AA tend to support each other emotionally and practically, which can be more effective than traditional one-on-one therapy for many individuals. Additionally, AA has been found to reduce healthcare costs due to fewer hospital visits and medical issues related to alcohol consumption.

What is not in debate is that it is the largest and oldest program with a singular purpose of helping people get sober at no cost. The steps are rooted in ancient wisdom and practices used throughout the world.

For many individuals, the cost of getting sober through a rehab center, therapist, or sober coach is out of reach. The 12-Step programs are mostly free, with the exception that meeting participants are asked to contribute a very small amount to pay for things like refreshments, rent for meeting rooms, and literature for hospitals and institutions. None of these fees are required for attendance, but it is common practice for a group and its members to be self-supporting. These programs are widely available—especially since the beginning of the Covid-19 pandemic—when thousands of meetings became available online worldwide, with 24/7 access.

Meetings occur in a variety of formats, so with a little persistence it's very likely you'll find one that works for you. Formats include topic discussion, book studies, speaker meetings, gender specific, and sexual orientation, to name a few. The reason there are so many different focus groups such as Alcoholics Anonymous, Narcotics Anonymous, Sex and Love Addicts Anonymous, Gamblers Anonymous, Overeaters Anonymous, and Debtors Anonymous is that there are different nuances to each of these groups, and it is helpful to talk to people who can understand and relate to those who are currently struggling with—or have struggled with—the same issues.

It is so helpful to hear from people who share similar feelings, talk about their struggles, what helped, and what life feels like on the other side. Some groups are faith-based and others are atheist based. But no matter what the problem is, the solution is the same. The solution is simple (not easy), it's spiritual (not necessarily religious), and it has nothing to do with the problem.

It's important to note that the success of any member depends heavily on a variety of factors, including the efforts of the individual, co-existing mental illness, the support of family and friends, and the degree to which they are ready to change—among others.

Let me give you a hint of what you might find if you decide to join a program and go through the process of the 12 Steps. My experiences relate to drugs and alcohol, so that's where the focus and majority of my examples are from, but you can literally replace any of those addictions with whatever you struggle with.

The purpose of the program is to help you gain access to a higher power so you can finally resolve the negative, addictive behaviors in your life. If you have not been able to reach your goals on your own, then spirituality—not necessarily religion—along with the support of the people at meetings, can help you achieve those goals.

Another more obvious benefit of sobriety? It could quite literally save your life. In addition to the previously stated health risks, according to the National Highway Traffic Safety Administration, 32% of all traffic fatalities are alcohol-related. For example, in 2022 alone there were around 13,600 fatalities due to drunk driving which translates to one death about every 39 minutes.

The good news is there is so much hope for change. If you begin attending meetings with an open mind and heart, it can renew a sense of hope and possibility for the future through spiritual experiences. There is nothing as convincing as having a personal experience that blows your mind. For those of us who have lost faith, we need evidence. We need to have our own experiences to convince us there might be another way of life. We need a sufficient substitute to replace the substances that no longer serve us.

I've had many spiritual experiences that left me absolutely in awe. These experiences feel like serendipitous events, "coincidences" so extraordinary I had no way to explain what had just happened, other than a loving energy that had a hand in guiding my experiences.

When I was pregnant with my second child, I had one of these spiritual experiences. My husband had been laid off from his job, and although he was working all kinds of odd jobs to make ends meet, it was obvious we were quickly going to fall short of paying the mortgage. At that time, I was running a daycare out of my home, but my belly had grown to the point where I was physically unable to work more than I already was. It was beginning to look like we were going to lose our house and I felt powerless to prevent it from happening. I had been sharing our predicament at meetings, and how I was managing my fears so I could stay sober. Other members of the community spoke up, sharing that they had the experience of losing their home and going bankrupt. And through it all they stayed sober. But, honestly, that sense of fellowship, of being implicitly understood didn't provide much comfort. I didn't want to go through all that! I kept asking myself, *What is the lesson here? What do I need to learn from this?* I finally realized that deep down, my self-worth was tied to my identity as a homeowner and financially responsible adult. That I held the belief that losing it all would mean I was not worthy as a person.

One day, the lesson finally sank in. It came to me as a feeling of deep knowing, that even if the worst happened and we lost everything, we would still be loved and we would be okay. My value as a person wasn't dependent on my financial status. The relief and peace I felt washed over me like a wave of gratitude.

It was Christmastime when all this was happening, and we were supposed to celebrate the holiday at my sister-in-law's home. She was extremely successful and had a huge, beautiful home, which made me feel even more ashamed that we didn't have the money to bring anything. She is one of the most gracious women I know, and all she wanted was to spend the holiday with us, but even so, I was still wrestling with feelings of shame and inadequacy.

On Christmas Eve, the day we were supposed to go celebrate with family, I walked out to my car in the rain, and that's when I saw it—a plastic bag tucked beneath my windshield wiper. It was a $100 gift card to the local grocery store. I instantly started sobbing with relief and gratitude. I had actual evidence that help would arrive. Standing there in the rain I truly understood that we were loved, and that our little family would be okay. And at least for this Christmas, I didn't have to show up emptyhanded.

To this day, I don't know who gave us the gift card but I know in my heart that this anonymous gift of hope was delivered by someone in the 12-Step program. My heart tells me this was God working in my life through people, which is usually how it goes for me. I don't pretend to fully understand my concept of God, but I believe that God can be found in the laws of the universe like gravity, karma, and law of attraction, but it is also personal. Personal in that it actually loves me as an individual and will do for me what I cannot do for myself.

For the sake of clarity, I want to provide a list of benefits provided by the 12-Step program and 12-Step community. There is a whole list of "Promises" in Chapter 6 of *Alcoholics Anonymous*. However, this is an addition to that list albeit not an exhaustive one.

i. You Can Overcome Alcohol and Regain Control of Your Life

This is the whole point—to quit the compulsive and destructive behaviors that are ruining your life. We do this by finding a power greater than ourselves and learning to regulate our emotions. We learn to take responsibility for our feelings and let go of responsibility that does not belong to us. Sobriety is just the beginning of personal and spiritual growth. When we learn to self-regulate by using the 12-Step process, we can apply the same principles to every aspect of our lives. This process will provide a way to process negative feelings to resolution so positive feelings can be cultivated. It leads to feelings of hope, freedom, peace, and happiness, as mood follows action.

ii. Your Life Will Have New Meaning and Purpose

Before I found the 12-Step community, I had so much guilt and shame over my past behavior. I felt deep remorse about the time I'd wasted, years lost to an obsession with alcohol I'd never get back and the pain I caused myself and others. What I learned is a new way to look at my past behavior. As it turns out, all the experiences I was so ashamed of could be used to help others. I became uniquely qualified to reach those who felt alone and isolated by being an example of a woman who has recovered from addiction.

I was told if I was going to remove drinking from my daily life, I would need to find a sufficient substitute. For me, this meant I would need new tools to help me manage my emotions. I needed relationships with like-minded people, and a community with the same purpose, to stay sober and help others achieve sobriety.

With this fresh perspective, I felt that my life had new meaning and purpose!

I'm not alone in this experience. It is very common that when this whole new world opens up for people, and finally there is a solution that dramatically transforms one's life in ways they never could have predicted, they often want to shout it from the rooftops. I can't tell you how many times I've heard people say, "The 12 Steps should be taught in schools!"

The program provides the coping skills most people never learn at home. It's a practical framework for managing emotions, gaining clarity, taking personal responsibility, finding community, and a place to do service and help others to recover from a potentially fatal disease.

iii. You Will Feel a Sense of Belonging

So many people feel as if they've never fit in anywhere. It is one of the most common experiences I've heard people share at meetings. The feeling of being uniquely different, isolated, and alone. These feelings are especially painful for those suffering with addiction. That's why having a community is a vital part of achieving recovery. 12-Step communities are made up of like-minded individuals, all dedicated to the pursuit of a common goal: to achieve sobriety, and to help others achieve it too.

It is important to find your people so you can feel seen, heard, and understood without judgment. By going to meetings, you will hear honest and vulnerable stories that will leave you astonished and surprised. At first, I was shocked to hear some of these stories. But as I listened, I heard people say things I was too afraid to admit, even to myself. Sometimes I'd hear things that I thought only *I* felt. I would think, *Yes that's true for me too!* I was relating and identifying on such a deeply profound level that I finally felt connected to the human experience.

Getting over the hurdle of going to your first meeting requires courage. Most people are scared to attend their first meeting, and that's normal. The tipping point is when the pain of not changing is worse than the pain of staying the same.

If you can, bring a friend so you feel safer. It will make it a lot easier to walk into that room for the first time. The truth is you *are* safe. You don't have to talk at your first meeting; you can simply observe until you feel comfortable enough to share.

When I was new to 12-Step meetings, I would sit in large crowds surrounded by people who knew each other. I watched as they would greet one another with love. They'd hug and smile and look so happy. After the meeting started, they'd tell stories of how some of the people in the room had helped them, and how it made a huge impact on their lives—which made me feel left out, but also envious, wanting what they had. I'd sit there and occasionally someone would introduce themselves to me.

One day, a well-respected woman approached me, stuck out her hand and said, "Hi, my name is CC. It's nice to meet you!" I stood there with my mouth open in awe. I'd heard her speak at many meetings and had been moved to tears by her stories, which had given me so much hope. From that day on, I made up my mind to start introducing myself to people at meetings. My line is always, "Hi, I'm Arlina, I haven't met you yet."

Although I didn't realize it at the time, I had fully accepted responsibility to feel connected. I wanted to become the person that made others feel welcome, even if they had been attending meetings longer than I had. I realized that there could be others in pain that day, who were unable to extend themselves in order to connect. Simply by saying hello, smiling, and acknowledging someone's presence, I could make a difference in someone else's life. By that simple act of service, I was rebuilding my self-esteem. Now I practice this skill intentionally, at every meeting I attend.

iv. You Will Find a New "Normal"

We change a lot while we are getting sober. In the program, we surround ourselves with other people who understand what it feels like to go through so many changes. We talk about all the new ideas we are learning as a way to make sense of it all. We talk about the struggle of knowing what we should do but repeating old patterns anyway. Sharing our challenging feelings is a practical way of processing them to resolution. Sometimes, just naming our fears takes the power out of them. It is a way to acknowledge and accept them, instead of avoiding or suppressing them.

For instance, when I first quit drinking there was a part of me that was sad to let go of alcohol. It was something that made me feel better, even if only temporarily. I knew it wasn't logical to be sad, but I just couldn't shake the feeling. I resisted telling anyone because I felt like there must be something really wrong with me. At meetings, I kept hearing things like "You're only as sick as your secrets." Finally, I found the courage to be honest about what I was feeling and shared it with my sponsor. She told me she had had those thoughts too! I felt so relieved. Her empathy was an antidote to my shame. Turns out, it's a common experience for people in recovery. It didn't mean there was anything wrong with me for having them. After our conversation, that feeling of sadness just kind of evaporated and I haven't felt that way since.

Another common experience to normalize is the feeling that life is suddenly boring. Without the highs and lows, life can feel a bit flat. It's important to understand that when you first quit drinking, your brain and digestive tract are healing from an oversaturation of dopamine and decreased serotonin production. Alcohol floods the brain with so much dopamine that it causes the brain to protect itself by removing dopamine receptors from cell membranes. It's called "receptor modulation."

That's why it takes more alcohol to feel the same high. As a result, when you stop drinking and artificially flooding your brain with dopamine, there is a period of time when life feels flat. Healing refers to the time it takes for the normal number of receptors to return to allow the uptake of dopamine.

Studies show that alcohol is also known to reduce the amount of serotonin produced in the gut, where 90% of all the serotonin in the body is produced. For some people, this decrease of serotonin can be the cause of depression.

Besides the neurochemistry that needs to return to normal, there's also the social aspect of recovery to consider. When we're drinking, we are reliant on alcohol to suppress our inhibitions so we feel more comfortable socializing. After we quit drinking, we need to relearn how to interact with others. It's normal to feel awkward and self-conscious about not drinking at first. With existing friendships, there is a period of adjustment especially if the friendship is centered on drinking. If you can find common ground in other activities, those friendships can transform and deepen. In social situations where you are interacting with new people, it's helpful to take the focus off of yourself and get curious about others so that conversations are easier.

Paradoxically, the fact that I had ruined all my friendships when I was drinking turned out to be lucky indeed as it forced me to start from scratch, to build a whole new network within the 12-Step community. My family was just happy to see that I was doing better so those relationships got better very quickly.

Here's the thing: a new normal imparts a sense of acceptance of how things are—not how we want them to be, or wish they were—of becoming comfortable with being uncomfortable at times. Or being comfortable not drinking in any situation and not feeling bad about it. Heck, I sometimes forget about drinking altogether! Others might have more awareness when alcohol or other addictive substances are present but when you do the work of recovery, it becomes part of the background, not the primary focus. A new normal can also mean having new friends who are on the same path. As a community, we joke that there's no such thing as small talk or oversharing in these circles. We become comfortable with expressing all our feelings. We know how to support each other, communicate effectively, and we show up for each other in astounding ways.

The 12-Step community is full of generosity and fellowship. There was a single mother of two who had recently lost her husband and then suffered a house fire, losing all her earthly possessions. It was amazing to see how the community rallied behind her. People organized a spaghetti dinner fundraiser, donated furniture, home goods, food, and temporary housing, in addition to offering emotional support. While she suffered a great loss, she knew she was loved and supported through it all.

I have also seen this community come together in times of illness. When a dear friend was diagnosed with cancer, everyone took turns bringing him food, taking him to the doctor, and organizing a fundraiser to help with his medical expenses. One member was a business executive in between jobs at the time and took it upon himself to manage our friend's medical care, working with doctors, nurses, and insurance companies to ensure he had the best possible care. I've never witnessed such an inspiring act of selfless service before. But in this community, that is "normal". It's just what we did for each other.

In early sobriety we often mourn our old way of life. Friends change, activities change, which can be lonely at first. But pretty soon, your calendar fills up quickly with meetings, sober parties, workshops, sober events, conventions, coffee with new friends, and so much more. Giving up drinking can feel like a loss at first, but it makes way for a whole new way of life, one which is as full and meaningful as you want it to be.

v. You Will Become the Best Version of Yourself

There is an old saying that when we know better, we *do* better. That is how we become the best versions of ourselves.

When negative thinking and behaviors are stripped away and replaced with new coping skills, it is finally possible to become the best version of yourself. Through the 12-Step process I learned that most of my dysfunctional behavior—such as codependency, substance-use disorder, and victim mentality—all stemmed from an inability to manage my emotions and resolve my negative feelings. I didn't learn many healthy coping skills when I was growing up, so I developed "survival skills," behaviors or obsessions that distracted me from the deep shame I often felt. My brain was literally trying to protect me by blaming others for my circumstances instead of taking responsibility for them, which often led to feelings of anger, frustration, and sadness.

Through recovery I learned that blaming others was choosing to give away my personal power to outside forces, whether a person, an institution, or a thing. When I learned how to take personal responsibility for my actions and let go of things I couldn't control, I got my power back and started making better choices. I learned we are all more powerful than we think, and that the first step is taking personal responsibility for our feelings. We may not get to choose what happens to us, but we do get to choose how we respond.

I had always been hugely dependent on external validation. I would try to look a certain way, or act a certain way, all in an effort to belong somewhere which is a normal human instinct for survival. In my case, I needed to practice extreme image management for others to love and accept me. At my core, I believed I was fundamentally not good enough, that there was something wrong with me, so I had to do twice as much as everyone else just to feel half as good. I became a people-pleaser, setting my own needs aside in hopes of receiving validation from others.

That way of life meant that my locus of control, or the source of my power, was located outside myself—and in the hands of others instead of my own. Any time there was conflict in my relationships, I was thrown onto an emotional rollercoaster ride. Once I took my power back by learning to validate myself and taking personal responsibility for my feelings, my life became more stable and outside influences had less of an effect on me.

This process has other benefits as well. It has allowed me to recognize when I'm comparing myself to others. As soon as I'm aware that I'm comparing, I change my focus to remember how far I've come and intentionally celebrate my own progress and achievement. Not that I don't still suffer from comparison on occasion, but it doesn't ruin entire days the way it used to.

vi. You Will Feel Better

The truth is you will feel everything better, the good and the bad. In the first few weeks of sobriety, I felt like one giant exposed nerve ending. It was as if the protective scab of drugs and alcohol was torn away, and any negative feeling was like sandpaper on an open wound. Thankfully, I had found the 12-Step community and had been introduced to women who had given me their phone numbers. They told me to call whenever I was in pain, feeling anxious, or just wanted to talk. It's hard to put into words how grateful I was for these new connections, but also how scared I was to call. I wanted to talk about my feelings, but I also didn't want to bother anyone. It was like being between a rock and a hard place.

Luckily, I had received what some people call the gift of desperation. I wanted to stay sober so badly that I put my fears aside, took a deep breath, and picked up the phone. What I learned was that it was a good idea to get into the habit of calling people when I felt stable, so that when the shit inevitably hit the fan and my brain was hijacked with emotions, I was already in the habit of reaching out.

This practice also kept me up to date with several members, so that if I did have an issue, I didn't have to spend a lot of time on the backstory—I could just get right into it and find some solutions. I dubbed this process "willingness calls." I ask all the women I work the program with to do at least one willingness call per day, especially in the beginning when you are building your support network. It's especially important to make willingness calls when you feel good, because unless you're already in the habit of calling it will be even harder to make calls when you don't feel good, and that's when we need connection the most. This is a program of action, and I have found this one practice to be the thing that has kept me sober during the most emotionally challenging times of my life.

vii. Your Relationships Will Improve

Healthy relationships are based on honesty, communication, and mutual respect. While in the throes of addiction, all that goes out the window and our relationships suffer as a result. To heal our relationships, we need an honest self-appraisal where we decide what we need to take responsibility for, and what we can let go of, without the skewed perspective of addiction. This can be achieved by working the 4th step.

By looking at your resentments and breaking them down to identify specific causes, you can identify how you were affected, your underlying fears, and—ultimately—what part you played in it all. A resentment is an unhealed wound we carry around like a pebble in a sack thrown over our shoulder. The weight might not be noticeable at first, but over time we collect so many pebbles the weight of the sack becomes crippling, and the pain becomes unbearable.

By listing your resentments, getting clear on their cause and effect, and sharing them with a sponsor, you can relieve yourself of this heavy burden. You can gain insight into taking responsibility for what you can control, let go of what you cannot, and avoid carrying those resentments in the future. As you notice how these resentments have affected your self-esteem, your relationships, and your sense of security, you will begin to develop self-compassion for having experienced so much pain without a way to resolve it. Without healthy coping skills, you developed dysfunction to manage the pain.

You will also see all the fears that came out of those resentments. Fears of not getting what you needed or of losing what you had. Fears that drove negative behavior patterns that caused emotional pain for you and others.

Perhaps the most important part of the 4th step is seeing the part you played in your own circumstances and how your behaviors affected others. When you can get to that place of empathy, and take responsibility for your part in things, your relationships often improve. Through the process of recovery, you also learn to rebuild your self-esteem by helping others. Through this process you can learn to love yourself, and then you can show up in relationships more honestly and authentically.

Now, I'm not saying this is an easy process. Not at all. It takes a tremendous amount of courage to practice this kind of honest self-examination. It is so humbling to see all the negative patterns of behavior! In *Alcoholics Anonymous* they call the underlying cause of these behavior patterns "character defects," such as pride, envy, jealousy, anger, sloth, lust, and greed. Natural instincts that are out of balance. I can honestly say the first time I truly faced these defects I hated them and felt deeply ashamed. Fortunately, I had a sponsor who was kind and compassionate, who often reminded me that I wasn't a bad person—I was doing the best I could with the survival skills I had, but that they were no longer serving me. Those words offered the perspective and context I needed to keep going.

Another sponsor once asked if I could love all of my unlovable parts. Immediately, I thought she was crazy. Of course I couldn't! There were parts of myself I downright hated. In my past, there were so many situations I didn't know how to handle. I was quiet when I should have spoken up or spoken up when I should have stayed quiet. I acted selfishly and hurt others, or completely abandoned myself to please them. I had made so many mistakes and had internalized the belief that I was defective. I didn't think I was smart enough or good enough to find love, or to even have friends.

For most of my life, I felt like I didn't belong anywhere so I would try extra hard to get people to like me, which is where my "people pleaser" tendencies come from. I was absolutely tortured by loneliness. It wasn't until I got sober and found the 12 Steps and the sober community that I began to understand how my past pain was creating dysfunction in my present-day relationships. My sponsor and friends treated my self-hatred with love and compassion. As they gave me context and perspective, I was able to receive love, see myself differently, and as a result I began making better choices. It changed how I interacted with people, who I allowed into my life, and allowed me to let go of people stuck in toxic behavior patterns I no longer wanted to participate in. Did I need to take responsibility and hold myself accountable? Absolutely! But that process was accompanied by love and support. I did not have to do it on my own. In fact, I couldn't have. I needed an outside perspective to help me see things clearly.

Emotion often clouds our perspective so we can't see things clearly. That's why when a friend presents a problem, the solution seems so obvious. We can see it clearly because we're unemotional. It might be helpful to note that feelings need to be validated before they can transform. Until you acknowledge a person's feelings by saying things like, "I can see how you'd feel that way," they often have trouble moving forward.

Everybody has a deep desire to be heard, seen, and understood. Ever get into a fight with someone and you started yelling because you felt like they weren't hearing you? Of course you have. It's because in that situation you need your feelings to be validated. A simple acknowledgement of understanding can diffuse the argument. Most people have the tendency to want to "fix" the other person by offering solutions, but that's not always helpful or even effective. Most people already know what they're supposed to do; they just need their feelings validated first.

Julie was a wise and gentle woman who sponsored me for a very long time. I would call her to complain about something and she would sit quietly until I was done venting. She'd calmly ask me what I needed. "Did you want to just vent, or would you like some feedback?" The first time she uttered those words, my jaw hit the floor. It had never occurred to me to simply ask for what I needed. What did I want from her?

At first, I had no idea, but after a few calls where she'd repeat the same question, I got more comfortable and began asking if I could vent for a few minutes before she offered suggestions or feedback. Up until that point, I had largely wanted sympathy or guidance on how to get someone to treat me the way I wanted them to. But the alternative Julie offered allowed me to begin noticing my feelings and the patterns of behavior I played out in response to those feelings.

Julie introduced me to the concept of making requests as opposed to demands, suggesting that I be open to outcomes, not attached to them. She helped me gain clarity on my feelings, and taught me how to deconstruct them in a way that helped me recognize where I was reacting to old wounds, not present circumstances. As I learned more and more about myself, I began to connect with parts of myself I had abandoned and denied. I learned that childhood trauma had caused me to disassociate and disconnect from myself, and that recovery was helping me to reconnect and resolve old pain. As I healed, I was better equipped to accept responsibility for my feelings, ask for what I needed, set boundaries where appropriate, and be a better friend and partner. There was a lot of trial and error, but also profound progress. My life looks nothing like it did when I first got sober, and it all started with changing my relationship with myself.

viii. You Will Stabilize Enough to Deal with Your Trauma

There is some debate in regard to whether you should stabilize first and then address trauma with a professional or do them at the same time. What I will say is that depends on the individual.

The first thing the 12-Step program helped me to resolve was the crisis around not being able to stop drinking and doing drugs. However, before I could do any intensive trauma work with a professional, I needed to allow my life to stabilize so the trauma work didn't trigger a relapse and cause more damage.

Completing the steps resulted in a complete overhaul of my life: I now had a solid support system, skills I used to manage my emotions, tools for regular self-care, and a much healthier self-esteem.

The steps were a practical way to sort through my emotional baggage. This process allowed me to let go of what wasn't mine so that I could bear the weight of what was.

My sponsor was gentle and compassionate, and helped me to see the part I'd played in every resentment I had, so I could recognize my patterns of behavior. She helped me to gain empathy for the people I hurt, gain clarity on why I reacted to certain situations, and taught me how to process my negative emotions. I learned to take responsibility for my actions and humbled myself to make amends so I could feel free. It was terrifying at times but cleaning up my side of the street cleared my conscience and left me with a sense of freedom I had never experienced. That's when the promises outlined in *Alcoholics Anonymous* started to come true for me. The guilt and shame I'd been carrying largely dissolved through this process.

Healing emotional pain has been an evolution for me. Going to meetings helped me to get comfortable with being vulnerable and sharing my thoughts, feelings, and experiences. Working with my sponsor helped me to feel safe in sharing the specifics of my emotional pain, and I received emotional support to face my fears. From there, I was encouraged to seek professional help to deal with the underlying trauma that contributed to my addictions. By healing my trauma, I am less reactive and now manage my emotions more effectively.

The vast majority of those who suffer with addiction have underlying trauma. I was in that category, too. When I was five years old, I was sexually abused by a neighbor's older child. The abuse happened repeatedly, and it went on for several years. The timeframe is fuzzy as I was so young but one thing I'm sure of is that it changed the trajectory of my life. The abuse fundamentally changed the course of my life because it happened while my identity was still being formed. It affected how I felt about myself, and what kind of person I thought I was.

Those experiences not only robbed me of my innocence; they robbed me of my voice. As I grew up, I remember being extremely uncomfortable when I was placed in situations where others wanted something from me and I didn't know how to say no. I didn't know how to speak up for myself and set firm boundaries. I just wanted to be liked. During that period, I was afraid to tell my mother what was happening; I thought she would be angry with me . My instincts were right.

One day she walked in on it happening and she completely freaked out. She got very angry and started yelling at us. There was shoving and crying. Feelings of shame, humiliation, and embarrassment washed over me. The worst part was that in that one moment I felt as if my mother hated me, as if some ugly hidden truth about me had been exposed. I'll never forget the look of disgust on her face. That one experience profoundly destroyed my self-esteem and self-worth.

What I learned after a lot of therapy and reading many self-help books, is that I'd developed certain survival skills to cope with what had happened to me—among them denial, dissociation, and detachment. I buried my feelings about the abuse deep inside, but they were never really gone. It was like a barrel of toxic waste that leached poison into every area of my life in the form of fear.

My whole life I had a deep-seated belief that there was something wrong with me, and that I'd need to work hard and achieve big things in life in order to overcome that defectiveness. I eventually used drugs and alcohol to numb those feelings of inadequacy, but I had other issues, too. Workaholism became another coping strategy later in life. For as long as I could remember, I'd always been a hard worker, holding down multiple jobs, but deep down I hated who I was, so I'd never allow myself to reach my goals, and self-sabotage became a consistent pattern in my life. I'd either quit working toward my goals or I would spread myself so thin that it was impossible to excel at any one thing.

In *What Happened to You?* Dr. Bruce D. Perry explains the effect trauma often has on the developing brain of a child and discusses how it impacts neurological development and behavioral patterns. The result of trauma is different for everyone. Some people develop hypersensitivity to pain and are labeled "overly sensitive" or are accused of being "drama queens." Others live in a chronic state of hypervigilance to avoid being hurt, which presents as being defensive and reactive. The good news is that there are many treatments available now that can help those afflicted effectively heal from traumatic events.

I have undergone many kinds of therapy myself including EMDR, Cognitive Behavioral Therapy, Internal Family Systems, and Process Therapy. I have used somatic practices like Emotional Freedom Technique, which is tapping, breathwork, yoga, and Reiki. I have practiced meditation for years in groups and on my own. I have also participated in many workshops on personal growth. These are all different modalities for healing that contribute to altering my Default Mode Network. I can now respond to challenging situations in a reasonable way rather than reacting to triggers that once hijacked my emotions.

ix. You Will Have Spiritual Experiences

Even through my religious baggage, my skepticism and doubt, I've had many transformational experiences that I cannot explain away with logic. These experiences feel so magical, so deeply personal, that I can only attribute them to a spiritual experience.

What is a spiritual experience? Well, for me, it's a feeling of serendipity and connectedness to people and to the natural world. It feels deeply personal and meaningful. These experiences often happen when I'm at the point of giving up. Then, out of the blue, something happens that gives me hope—like when my heart is hurting, and I go to a meeting and someone says the exact thing I need to hear. This has happened more times than I can count. Or, for instance, at those moments when I have the courage to share something about myself that feels shameful and instead of disdain, it is met with empathy and compassion. That feeling of connectedness and belonging gives me hope that maybe I'm not alone, and that these unbearable feelings won't last forever. A spiritual experience is undeniable and when it happens to you, you just know; even if you only realize it in hindsight. It's like falling in love. Someone can explain to you what it feels like, but you don't really understand until you experience it for yourself.

12

The Pre-Game: What to Know Before You Start

i. Read the Literature for Yourself

Everyone has a unique perspective on the literature, and it can be very helpful to speak with others at meetings to get a deeper understanding. However, that does not mean you should solely rely on what other members say. There is no person who represents the organization. For instance, there are some old-timers who say things like "We don't take nothin' no matter what!" Guess what? That's not the official message from the organization. In fact, there's a pamphlet sponsored by AA on the topic of medication, which states "No A.A. member should "play doctor"; all medical advice and treatment should come from a qualified physician."

The point here is that there are a lot of common ideas circulating around meetings that are not sanctioned by the organization, which is why you will need to read the literature.

ii. A Fresh Perspective and New Context

Having a balanced perspective and context around challenging ideas is the difference between quitting early and finishing the steps. If you're at the point where you're considering a 12-Step program, take a step back to consider what your mindset is. It might be time to set aside your fears and reconsider some of your most basic assumptions.

At the beginning of this journey, your mindset is likely to be in defense mode and crisis mode at the same time. That fear will be at an all-time high, triggering cognitive bias—meaning we only accept information that is in line with what we already believe and reject any information that isn't. This bias causes the "contempt prior to investigation" mindset which is the practice of making sweeping judgments based on superficial information acquired secondhand, rather than evaluating your results based on your own personal experience.

Here's the deal: Your way of thinking about quitting and the actions you've been taking up to this point are not working. How do I know this? Because you wouldn't be reading this book if they were. But it's not really your fault, and here's why. When you were a child, you were influenced by the people who raised you and the people around you on a daily basis. If you experienced any kind of trauma—from small traumas to the extreme—you developed coping skills to survive, in the form of toxic behavioral patterns. For instance, if you were in emotional pain and were not comforted, or worse yet, if you were physically isolated, you learned that when you are in pain you need to isolate. Maybe that pattern helped you to survive, but it doesn't lead to living a healthy lifestyle or forming secure adult relationships.

Although the unhealthy behavioral patterns aren't your fault, it is your responsibility to heal them, to manage your emotions, and create the life you want. So, to change your experience, you have to be willing to reconsider your perspective. It is our emotions and thinking that need to be healed. We make decisions emotionally and justify them logically. The influx of new information, new evidence, and new experiences is the pathway to change our thinking, and it is how healing occurs. There is nothing more convincing than evidence and personal experiences. That is one of the biggest benefits of the 12-Step program. At meetings, you will hear the experiences of others firsthand, and see people change in real-time.

iii. Beware of "Contempt Prior to Investigation"

Does it make sense to trust the judgment of someone you do not know or respect to determine whether this is a viable program for you? Of course not! Instead, I propose that you investigate, have your own experience, and then come to your own conclusions. Just like any organization with millions of members, most of whom struggle with a degree of mental illness, there are many people who make mistakes as they are healing. Maybe these are the people who have turned you off from trying it for yourself.

What is important to note here is that for every negative example, you will find many positive ones. My suggestion would be to talk to the people who have what you want, ask them what they do, and then try it for yourself. Keep trying until you find something that works for you.

If you are considering going to a 12-Step meeting, begin the process with the mindset of experimentation. Take the suggestions offered to you, apply them to your life, and only after completing ALL the steps can you come to a conclusion based on your own experience.

iv. The First Meeting

The first meeting is always the hardest. It might feel intimidating to walk into a room of people, not knowing what to expect. Bringing a friend for moral support helps a lot. You might be afraid you will see someone you know. If you do, just remember that they're there for the same reason you are. But the truth is, every meeting is different. If you're afraid to share, you can simply say it's your first meeting and you're there just to listen. You could also try a speaker meeting for your first time, which is where one person shares their story for the duration. You can find those meetings by calling your local central office or looking them up online. Most people at meetings are welcoming and friendly. If they aren't, don't be discouraged—just try another meeting.

v. You Might Feel like an Outsider at First

When you start going to meetings, you'll notice that some people already know each other. They might get locked into conversation and not notice new people. Try not to take it personally. I recommend that you go to the same meeting every week, so that you start to get to know people, and they get to know you too. You might even volunteer for a service position. Service positions include setting up, bringing coffee or snacks, finding speakers, or running the meeting. Those positions will not only get you to the meeting, but in the process you'll get to know other members better and you'll generally start feeling a part of the group. You get out of meetings what you put into them, so step outside your comfort zone and invest a little bit of time and effort into a group you like.

vi. Not Everyone is Safe

Common sense tells us that in any large organization, especially one centered on addiction, there will be people who are not safe in terms of physical or emotional safety.

There will be people at meetings who don't really want to be there. For instance, the legal system sometimes sends people to AA who have no interest in recovery, and who are there only out of obligation. They are there to get their court card signed to get the judge off their back or avoid legal consequences. Some of these individuals may even prey on vulnerable members. I'm not saying this to scare you away from meetings, but to encourage you to exercise a bit of caution.

A lot of people with alcohol-use disorder also have other unhealthy coping skills, such as codependency, sex and love addiction, and/or workaholism. When I was a young woman new to the program, I was told to stick with the women and to avoid dating in the first year to keep my focus on recovery. There is a term called "13 Stepping," which refers to the fact that some people will try and date newcomers—which is a terrible idea, considering that newcomers are often emotionally vulnerable, and entering these relationships can easily trigger a relapse. Socializing in a group setting is much safer for all involved. Watch and listen, then pick your people carefully. I highly recommend same-sex meetings in the beginning, if they are available in your area.

vii. You Don't Have to Share if You Don't Want to

At some meetings, you might get asked to introduce yourself or share. It's okay to say, "I'm just listening today," or "I'm going to pass for now, thanks."

I will say that sharing in a general way is a great way to process negative feelings. You probably don't want to get too specific or go into great detail, but sharing allows others to get to know you and helps you to feel connected to the group.

You could also attend "speaker meetings," where there is one person who tells their story and nobody else shares. You can simply go and listen until you feel comfortable enough to try a meeting where you can share.

viii. Nobody Can Run You Out of a 12-Step Meeting

The only requirement for membership is a desire to stop drinking. Period. There is no boss, president, or leader who can tell you what to do or what you should think. There is no one person who speaks for every 12-Step program, meeting, or community. If you attend meetings, you will hear many strong opinions—some of which may cause you to feel angry or uncomfortable. You might even hear many of the same ideas from multiple members of the organization, but just because they say it doesn't mean they speak for AA as a whole.

This is why it's so important to study the literature yourself and develop your own understanding of what it means. It takes courage to stay open-minded. If you hear things you don't agree with at meetings, you can choose to talk things over with trusted friends, or your sponsor to get their perspective. Remember, the goal is to find the context and perspective that will allow you to make progress and complete the steps.

ix. Not All Meetings are Created Equal

If you have a negative experience at a meeting, there are a few options to consider. You can try attending that particular meeting one more time, just to see if your initial assessment was correct. Some meetings are fun and lighthearted, but others are much "heavier". Different members show up at each meeting, so you just need to find one or two people you connect with. It's also possible that you might need to attend a few meetings to just get comfortable. The other option is to **find another meeting.** You can literally go online to AA.org and look up meetings in your area through the app, appropriately named, "Meeting Guide." You can also try online meetings. If you find a meeting that feels like home, you're in the right place. Again, meetings are not the program, but they are an important part of working the steps.

x. Sponsors are Not Professional Therapists

AA is a peer support program. Sponsors are not to be treated as therapists who are trained professionals legally bound to maintain confidentiality.

The advantage of a sponsor is that they will spend a lot more time with you, and they'll do it for free. A lot of people talk to their sponsors on a daily basis. Some sponsors even make themselves available day or night in case you need to call them.

Just keep in mind that sponsors make mistakes, like everyone else, and because of this sometimes sponsors will say things that are wrong or inappropriate. Some sponsors can even be controlling or demanding. If this occurs, you have every right to find a new sponsor. Just don't give up on the process because of one person's actions.

xi. Judgmental Old-Timers

You should know from the outset that you will on occasion run across some crotchety old-timers who think they know everything and have no problem telling everyone their opinion. This will be a great time to practice patience! Just because a member has maintained their sobriety for many years does not mean they are mentally and emotionally well. Their thinking can be outdated, they can be abrasive, and occasionally do more harm than good.

What's important to know is that such individuals do not speak for the entire organization. Nobody does. If they say something hurtful, forgive and let it go. Instead, focus on connecting with your people.

xii. There's So Much 12-Step Jargon!

For instance, you'll hear people talk about, "The Big Book," which is the nickname for the basic text, *Alcoholics Anonymous*. Or you might hear paradoxical phrases like "surrender to win," or "you have to give it away to keep it," or "pride in reverse." Don't worry if you don't really get what people are talking about at first. You can always ask but just keep in mind everyone will have a different answer and that's okay. You will start to make sense of it all after a while.

xiii. The Thing About Anger

"Anger is an acid that can do more harm to the vessel in which it is stored than to anything on which it is poured." —Mark Twain

In the book, *Twelve Steps and Twelve Traditions*, it states that alcoholics are not capable of handling anger and that it should be left to people who are better qualified. I believe the point of this idea is to encourage people in recovery to resolve their anger rather than hang onto it.

While anger can often be precarious territory, in the right context it can also be a catalyst for change. I'd like to reframe the idea that people struggling with addiction are not capable of handling anger and instead introduce the idea that when anger is confronted with compassion, it can be processed to resolution.

Tara Brach—a psychologist, author, and teacher of meditation— explains that anger is often a sign of an unmet need. When our needs aren't met, we can shift our thinking to identifying those needs in order to find ways they can be met either within ourselves, or by seeking help from a licensed therapist.

13

Handy Tips for the Journey

i. How to Find a Healthy 12-Step Group

To find a healthy group requires some trial and error. The meetings I love most are ones with members that make newcomers feel welcome. They give out books, phone numbers, and offer up recommendations to other meetings they'd personally found helpful and remember people's names. Healthy groups start on time, end on time, and have clear boundaries. Members will gently remind each other to adhere to the 12 traditions. They cultivate a sense of belonging and safety for each other.

In healthy groups, you hear people share on the topic, read, or quote the literature, and relate it to their own personal experience. They say things like, "this is what it means to me," or "I found this to be helpful." They share their pain with the group, but also talk about solutions for it—instead of simply dwelling on their problems.

There will be a balance of problems and solutions. Healthy groups are not solely focused on the negative, but also the positive side of recovery. We often say that we're not a glum lot, that we are a group of people who insist on having a good time, and I have found that to be true. We often joke around before, during, and after meetings.

There is always some milestone celebration, birthday, picnic or BBQ, convention, or event to attend.

But not every meeting is full of fun and laughter. People go to meetings to share their feelings, and to process some heavy experiences along the way. Just by showing up and listening, you are providing a service, an act of love and kindness.

The meetings I have enjoyed the most were ones where I left feeling relieved and hopeful, where the exact solution for my pain was offered up. I have noticed the meetings I get the most out of are ones at which I had an opportunity to share. Even on those rare occasions where I didn't get to share or resonate with the topic, there was usually at least one comment or story that saved the meeting for me and made it worth my time.

ii. A Sponsor's Role and How to Find a Good One

AA has a well-written pamphlet on sponsorship that you can find on their website.

The purpose of a sponsor is to take you through the 12 Steps; and share their experience, strength, and hope with you. Sponsors aren't professional counselors, therapists, or doctors. They shouldn't give advice or interfere with medications prescribed by a physician.

They are not responsible for your recovery. It is up to you to reach out to them, set appointments with them, and do the 12-Step work they ask you to do. They are not to be treated like banks, or a taxi service. They are also not your boss or parent, nor do they have any authority over you whatsoever. If you are not willing to trust them or take their suggestions, you might consider finding someone who is a better fit. There is a saying in the rooms that, "there is a wrench for every nut." So, if you don't think you have the right sponsor, keep looking. Of course, if you go through a dozen sponsors in short order, you might need to look inward to discover what is preventing you from taking their suggestions. Many newcomers self-sabotage out of fear. The good news is that when you're ready, you'll do the work.

Since getting sober in 1994, I've had six sponsors. Each of these beautiful women took time out of their busy lives to talk with me, to share their experience and wisdom—but mostly, they loved me. They'd ask me to do some writing exercises, we would read the literature together, I would share what I wrote, and we'd talk about it. We'd also discuss the challenges I was having that week, and I'd ask for their feedback.

In connecting with the right sponsor, I've been told over the years to look for someone who had what I wanted, and then emulate them. I would go to many of the same meetings regularly and pay attention to the women who said things I resonated with. The women I was attracted to were those who were gentle, calm, and wise; who had completed the steps and who routinely performed acts of service in the group.

iii. How to Build Your Support System

Building a support system of trusted friends and allies who are on the same path as you is of utmost importance, people who will understand what it feels like to have cravings, what it's like to feel awkward in social settings without alcohol, and those who can relate to the wild range of emotions that comes with getting sober. There's just something comforting about not feeling alone during this transition. I refer to this as a "system," as it's not the greatest idea to depend on just one or two people. Everyone is busy these days, so if you need someone to talk you off the ledge, you will fare better if you have several people you can call.

If you are ready to make your sobriety a priority and build a support system, I suggest you perform a series of "willingness calls"—choose a few people to call weekly, moving outside your comfort zone to build new connections. It's like a check-in call where you ask how they are doing; you share something that's going on with you, and maybe make plans to go to a meeting together or meet up for coffee. That's it! If you don't have a lot of time to chat, or don't want to get stuck on the phone, you can simply start the conversation with, "I only have a few minutes, but I wanted to check in on you."

The whole purpose of these willingness calls is to get comfortable connecting with others, to ease into this process by calling when you're not in a moment of crisis. You need to get into the habit of calling your people when you feel stable, as it's incredibly hard to call when you're in emotional pain, unless you are already in the habit of doing so. And, if you are already up to date with someone, you can get right into the solution instead of spending a lot of time on the backstory. If you are current with several people and one person isn't available, you have others you can call.

Don't be discouraged if it takes some time to find your support system. Expect to reach out to a handful of people. Some won't call you back. They are not your people, and that's okay. You might decide that someone you contact initially isn't a good fit for you. That's okay too. The point is to keep trying because we all need a support system.

One of the most common objections to this request is "But I don't want to bother anybody." Here is the truth: You are doing them a favor by giving them an opportunity to be of service. We must give it away to keep it, so you are actually helping them stay sober! Also, I have had so many magical conversations just by reaching out and checking in on people. There have been so many times when I called and the person on the other end immediately exclaimed, "I'm so glad you called; I was feeling so off today, and this really helped!"

You might think you will call someone before you drink, but if you haven't been practicing, remember this: "We do not rise to the level of our expectations. We fall to the level of our training." —Archilochus, Greek Soldier, 650 BC

So where do you start? You start by going to meetings and asking for phone numbers, which is a common practice. Many meetings will have lists of members posted who are willing to take calls. I would recommend texting first to let them know where you got their number, so your call doesn't go straight to voicemail. Then ask if they have a couple of minutes to talk. It's important to talk on the phone, not just text. It doesn't have to be a long call, but it can be. Every person and every situation is different, but the idea is to start making new friends. Alcoholism is a disease of isolation, and connection is the cure.

PART 3

Overcoming Common Barriers to Entry – Myths, Misperceptions, and Truths About 12-Step Programs

14

Can't I Just Learn To Moderate?

If you are still thinking you can learn to moderate your alcohol intake, *Alcoholics Anonymous* suggests trying some controlled drinking to help you decide. For instance, try to have just one or two drinks, but if you end up drunk at the end of the evening that is a sign you cannot moderate. If you have enough evidence from past experiences that you are unable to stick to a moderate drinking plan consistently, the suggestion is to abstain from drinking entirely—especially when working the steps with a sponsor.

I personally believe you must conclude that you cannot drink in moderation before you embrace a life of abstinence. It's a question that must be fully answered to the depths of your soul in order to embrace the program. What has worked for me since 1994 is to focus on a decision to remain alcohol-free, by taking it one day at a time. To be transparent, I haven't thought about it in years but it was a mindset that helped me get through the beginning phase. And don't worry about future celebrations like weddings and holidays, or how you'll get through tough events like death, divorce, or extreme crisis without alcohol. You can't drink today for tomorrow's events anyway. You can, however, decide that just for today—or just for the next hour or the next minute—you are not going to drink.

Everyone in this position will ask themselves, *Is my drinking bad enough that I have to quit?* But that's not the question that will lead to a decision. That question is like taking a ride on a merry-go-round. It's a distraction of highs and lows that just takes you in circles.

The real question is, *Do the benefits of drinking outweigh the consequences?* That, my friend, is the pivotal question with which to begin.

Exercise:

Take a minute to write a pros and cons list about what might happen if you were to continue drinking. Be as honest as you can with this list, as finding positive alternatives will be the next step. And over the next few days, think hard about the cons list. If you still are drinking, be fully present in the consequences or after-effects of your drinking. For example:

- How does my body feel right now?
- Am I closer to the important people in my life? Or has drinking created a wedge between us?
- To what degree do I feel guilt and shame about my recent behavior?
- Is drinking in alignment with my authentic self?
- Is drinking interfering with reaching my goals?

This exercise can help you see the impact of your drinking more clearly. What does it have to cost you before you decide it is bad enough to quit? What if you decide that you and your loved ones deserve better? Spend some time writing about the life you would like to have, and how alcohol might be interfering with creating that life for yourself.

Listen, I get it. It's not easy to make the decision to quit. It took me two years of experimenting with moderation before I finally found the willingness to let it go. One obstacle was the common tendency to compare myself to others who were worse off. It's tempting to look at those who have lost everything and convince us we're fine because we haven't reached those depths yet. I haven't destroyed my life like those people who have multiple DUIs, spent time in prison, lost jobs, wrecked relationships, ruined their health etc. We have all seen drunk and homeless people on the street and thought, *Yeah, that's what an alcoholic is. They definitely need help.* It's human to feel at least a little superior to any extreme, to believe your own drinking isn't that bad in comparison.

In reality, your drinking may *not* be as bad as those who have lost everything. Maybe you're just sick of the hangover hamster wheel or waking up at 3:00 am every night because you drank too much before bed. Maybe you're simply sick and tired of feeling sick and tired. Or sick of feeling angry, lonely, and empty inside—where the only perceived solution to those feelings is to have another drink. Maybe you're tired of hearing the stories of what you did or said the night before, and the shame that routinely follows suit. Or maybe you're tired of having to apologize to angry family members yet again, not knowing if they're being overly dramatic because you can't remember exactly what you did to make them so angry and upset. In any case, these are all signs that your drinking is, in fact, bad enough to stop.

From an outsider's perspective, it's not hard to see when someone's drinking has become problematic. However, we often don't have the same awareness once we start drinking, which can fool us into believing our behavior hasn't changed that much—or, at least, that we're fooling everyone. It's challenging to objectively see ourselves with clarity. How can we? Our brains are literally impaired while under the influence, and the parts of our brain used to process information are compromised. Think about the times when you were sober and other people were drunk and acting the fool. Were you embarrassed for them? Concerned? Is it possible your friends and family have felt the same about you? If you've ever woken up and thought, *I'm never doing that again!* this could be your sign that it's time to stop.

15

AA? No Way! My Drinking Isn't THAT Bad!

When considering how to quit drinking, AA might seem like a big leap. Especially if you aren't convinced that your drinking is "bad enough." After all, you still have a good job, you're financially stable-ish (who doesn't have room for improvement here!?), you still have your family, and you've never gotten arrested for drunk driving. So, you might be tempted to think your drinking isn't bad enough for AA which is fair. It's a common misperception that you must be a daily drinker or have lost everything and/or be on the brink of insanity or something equally catastrophic to join AA. Not true. The truth is anyone could benefit from going through the 12-Step process. It is a very practical way to practice self-examination, optimize personal growth, improve relationships, and be a part of a community.

Underneath the idea: *My drinking isn't bad enough to join AA* begs the question: *Is what I'm doing to stop drinking working for me?*

Take a few minutes to list all the ways you have tried to stop drinking. Then simply look at the effects. Over the years that I've been sober, I've heard so many methods people used to try to quit. Everything from multiple rehabs, reading every recovery memoir, listening to every podcast, going to church, various 30-day challenges, a taper-down approach, switching to non-alcoholic beer or wine, and I've even heard of people taking medications like Antabuse, and still drinking. Some of these approaches work for some people. However, if you haven't been able to stop, or stay stopped, then you have your answer. It's time to try something different.

In truth, you don't have to compare your drinking to that of others to join the program. Your feelings and experiences are valid enough. You don't have to hit rock bottom. You can stop wrestling with alcohol if you want to. There's no shame in that. In fact, it takes a tremendous amount of courage to let go of alcohol and embrace a new way of life. Especially since we live in a drinking culture where we are actually *expected* to drink. People drink at work, at parties, in mom groups, at church, camping, after marathons…everywhere. It's the only drug that you have to explain why you are NOT doing it. It's actually such an incredible act of courage and rebellion to not drink!

The thing is, issues with alcohol show up differently for everyone who struggles—no matter where they fall on the addiction spectrum. Someone with alcohol-use disorder can be a daily blackout drinker or an occasional binge drinker—it just depends. It's not about how much you drink; it's about what happens when you do . When I drank, I would say things I normally wouldn't say, like tell my friends what was wrong with them or how much I hated their boyfriends. I was totally unfiltered. But that's what happens when you drink. The frontal lobe of your brain responsible for social appropriateness is the first to go offline. People often say that alcohol is a truth serum, but really it's just spewing impulsive, unfiltered, incomplete thoughts. We needlessly hurt the ones we love when we drink and everyone, including ourselves, suffers.

We also do things under the influence we normally wouldn't do. I used to drink and then drive home, thinking I was fine. It's a miracle I never hurt anyone or myself. I would go out partying and wake up with strangers. I would get overly emotional and cry in public, then feel totally humiliated the next day. I think about how the people around me must have felt about me. How they must have lost respect for me and felt embarrassed for me. It's no wonder that at the end I had very few friends and my career was going down the toilet.

If drinking causes you shame, humiliation, and sickness—or damages your relationships and reputation—maybe it's time to find another way to relax, socialize, or deal with stress.

I just want to take a moment to point out that addiction is not a moral issue. Experts will disagree on what it is exactly, but they commonly agree that it's a biological, psychological, and I would dare to take it a step further—spiritual issue. Our complete makeup involves body, mind, and spirit. When one system is affected, so are the others.

Addiction can happen to anyone and in fact it does. In 12-Step meetings, you will see all walks of life: doctors, clergy, men, women, young, old, rich, and poor. People from all religions, from all over the world, from every kind of family, from healthy to dysfunctional, from every socioeconomic background. If you drink long enough and often enough, you will develop alcohol-use disorder.

We're not bad people trying to get good; we are hurt people trying to medicate the pain. By medicating the emotional pain, we detach from it instead of resolving it which causes the pain to persist. If the coping skill is to medicate with drugs and alcohol, the addiction escalates.

It's human instinct to distract ourselves from emotional pain. In my case, I had become so numb to my own pain I didn't even realize how bad things were. I had totally lost perspective and had grown so accustomed to the drama that routinely played itself out in my life that it seemed normal to me.

There's an idea called shifting baseline syndrome that explains how otherwise reasonable people fall into these dysfunctional patterns. It is an evolutionary concept that harkens back to the past, when times were difficult due to famine, drought, or war, for example.

The shifting baseline refers to the fact that when things get worse, we get used to it and it becomes normalized. Our brains do this out of self-preservation to relieve stress. It prevents us from getting so despondent over things we can't control that we give up. After all, our brains are designed to help us survive, which is why we often live in dysfunctional behavior patterns. But we don't deserve condemnation for this; we deserve compassion. After all, if we truly had healthier coping skills we would have used them.

We discuss shifting baseline syndrome routinely in the 12-Step rooms by referring to it as "seeking lower companionship." For instance, when I was still drinking Tuesday nights were dollar drink night at a local restaurant. I would grab a friend who liked to drink like I did, and we'd go get really drunk. The funny thing is that crowd was rough! I mean, who goes out in the middle of the week to get drunk?! It's ironic that I thought I was better than those people when I was doing the same thing as they were. But that's what I mean about seeking lower companionship. I was socializing with people I didn't respect because they were the only ones who thought it was okay to get wasted on a Tuesday night.

Now I understand why we do that. It's so we don't feel as bad about our drinking in comparison. Over time, we don't recognize how bad our drinking has become. Other people in our lives can see it clearly, but in the depths of our addiction we tend to see those people as controlling or judgmental. We dismiss their concerns out of fear because we are afraid of losing the one coping mechanism we have come to depend on. No judgment here; we do what we must to survive. We are created to survive through belonging.

For many in the sober-curious phase, there comes a time when they begin to realize they are unable to control their alcohol usage—whether the amount, frequency, or occasion. At some point they recognize they have lost the ability to choose whether or not to drink. Drinking becomes a *must*. If that sounds like you, this could be the moment when you find the willingness to give the 12 Steps a try.

The good news is that the program is about discovering a sufficient substitute. A substitute that quite literally fills the void quitting drinking leaves. Over the three decades I've been attending meetings, the most common conclusion I hear is, "I had no idea that this is what recovery is. If I'd only known, I would've started a long time ago and saved myself so much heartache."

16

Admit I'm an Alcoholic? No Thanks!

First, let's address the word "alcoholic." It typically carries a negative connotation. Our minds conjure up the worst images of people who are destroying their lives and are dangerous, selfish, mean, and insane. Who would want to identify with that?

Not wanting to call yourself an alcoholic is a very real and valid issue. Truthfully, it is outdated language. Psychology has evolved a tremendous amount since *Alcoholics Anonymous* was first published in 1939. The Diagnostic and Statistical Manual of Mental Disorders (DSM5) used to diagnose mental health disorders now uses the term 'alcohol-use disorder.' It was changed because to some 'alcoholic' is stigmatizing and creates a barrier for people to get help.

However, for a lot of people who have joined AA the word has been redefined and holds special meaning that is useful for them. There is a way to temper the idea of identifying as an alcoholic, that makes the rest of the program easier to swallow.

The solution here is to redefine what the word means. An alternative definition includes someone who comes to accept that they are not able to manage their drinking effectively. At some point in trying to manage my drinking, I realized my body does not process alcohol like some other people. Drinking caused me to black out. It kicked in this desire for more once I started. I didn't drink every day, but when I drank it was almost always to excess—even when I swore to myself I'd only have one.

After I got sober and attended meetings regularly, I began to see the word and the people associated with it in a different light. Most of the people at meetings looked like everyone else. There were representations from all walks of life. More importantly, they wore the label like a badge of honor. For me and many others, the label of "alcoholic" has come to mean a person of courage who was strong enough to face reality, to face their pain by practicing self-reflection, and to choose themselves over a glass of poison. Alcoholics are rebels who defy the immense social pressure to drink. I see people who identify as an alcoholic as a kindred soul. With a single word, I know that they are like me: fighting the good fight to stay sober and dedicated to personal growth and helping other people get sober when they can.

What you hear at meetings from other members about what has to be done to stay sober varies greatly. It's not uncommon to hear people say you "have" to admit you're an alcoholic, or you "have" to work the steps, that you "have" to accept a higher power etc. The truth is you don't "have" to do anything. The literature states that we only offer suggestions (albeit strong ones sometimes). The only requirement for membership is a desire to stop drinking .

Admitting that I was an alcoholic at the beginning of my sober-curious phase was difficult, to say the least. A lot of people resist it. I've heard from many people over the years that they only concluded they related to the idea of having alcoholism after hearing many stories at meetings, not at the start of their journeys.

Another point of contention is that you will hear people at meetings introduce themselves by saying something like, "My name is Mary, and I'm an alcoholic." The reason people introduce themselves in this way is out of a tradition that started back in the late 1930s when open meetings were established. Friends and family would often attend these meetings to support their friends and loved ones who were struggling. The idea was that people who wanted to stop drinking could bring someone so they'd feel more comfortable.

Doctors and clergy would routinely attend these meetings so they could recommend them to their patients and parishioners. With so many support people attending meetings and sharing, the people trying to quit were not being heard. At some point, it was determined that only people wanting to stop drinking—or "alcoholics"—should share their stories, so that's why we introduce ourselves the way we do. That's also a big reason why so many other recovery groups such as Al-Anon began, as it became clear early on that alcoholism is a family disease.

The moniker of "alcoholic" is not the only way people introduce themselves at meetings, but it's the most common. I've also heard people say, "My name is Mary, and I recovered from alcoholism" to avoid a label they are uncomfortable with. I've heard people say they are a recovered alcoholic, sober alcoholic, or a real alcoholic. The truth is there is no requirement to introduce yourself in a specific way. We are a group of people who hate to be told we HAVE to do something. That's almost a surefire way to get someone to do the opposite. There's a line in *Alcoholics Anonymous* that says "rebellion dogs our every step." The antidote to this rebellion is to take the pressure off by making suggestions rather than insisting everyone follow strictures that aren't in the "Big Book."

All that joining the program entails is simply showing up with a desire to stop drinking. Everyone must start at the beginning and get curious about their relationship with alcohol or other substances. Objective self-examination is the goal, as is releasing guilt and shame. This type of analysis leads to insights and wisdom into our behavioral patterns, and what drives us to act the way we do. When you first begin examining your relationship with alcohol, my suggestion would be to hold off on relying on your own interpretation of that word or other challenging concepts and listen to what others have to say about what it means to them.

17

Who Said I'm Powerless?

I've heard many times from people in alternative programs that this was the word that stopped them dead in their tracks. That it made them reject the possibility of 12-Step work, as they did not believe they were powerless over their lives. However, they are not looking at the complete phrase, which is admitting one's <u>powerlessness over alcohol</u>. While I would agree that no one is powerless in general, if they have lost the ability to choose whether they drink or not—or how much they drink—they *are* in fact powerless over alcohol.

I would argue that everyone is powerless over alcohol to some extent. The whole point of consuming alcohol is to change the way you feel, and alcohol has the power to do that. Biologically speaking, once a person has consumed alcohol they have kicked off a cascade of chemical reactions that physically change the way the brain functions. Once this chemical reaction starts, it cannot be reversed at will. Only time will allow the body to return to normal.

18

Isn't AA Just Religious Stuff?

This is also a valid concern, but it doesn't have to be a dealbreaker. There are people of faith and many who have no faith that have benefited from the program. All of these disparate groups have found a way to complete the steps. However, I will validate that if you already have a belief in God, the 12-Step process will be easier for you.

The Christian influence in the program is undeniable. While one of the founders, Bill W., was agnostic both he and the other founder, Dr. Bob, had previously been part of the Christian-based Oxford Group. They left to start Alcoholics Anonymous because they felt alcoholics had already experienced too much evangelical pressure and wanted to support people in finding their own higher power.

In some meetings, you will find that they still say the Lord's Prayer, the 7th step prayer, and the Serenity prayer. This was a huge barrier for me when I first joined, since I had so much religious trauma in my past and I know it's often a problem for others as well. An objection I hear repeatedly in one variation or another is, "If I have to pray to God, this isn't going to work for me."

Now, I'm not going to try to talk you out of your beliefs; rather just ask that you consider this question: Who gets to decide what that concept of God, or a "higher power," is for you? The short answer is *you*. It can only be you. In the beginning of this process, you get to find a concept that makes sense to you, to define what that word means to *you*. You can even borrow an acronym to start out with, like: God—Good Orderly Direction, Group of Drunks, or Great Outdoors.

Another important point to consider is that there is a difference between religion and spirituality. Religion refers to a specific set of beliefs, whereas spirituality involves the recognition of a belief or feeling that there is a greater universal energy that is Divine in nature.

Here's my personal, admittedly limited, concept of God. I know as soon as I write it down, I'll want to amend it but this is the general idea. God is both universal and personal. It's the source of universal power that always *was* and always *will be*. It created the laws of the universe: gravity, karma, the law of attraction, space, time, and physics. Yet this power is also loving and personal to me, like that of a parent/child relationship, a loving energy that is special to me, but also to all sentient beings. It resides inside of me, but also surrounds me in everything. Aligning me with a creator whose intention is to support my soul's growth and evolution which co-creates my reality. It's an experience of deep love and connectedness. This power manifests through serendipitous events and through the people who enter my life in ways I can't always explain with my head, but that I can feel in my heart.

I don't see this higher power as having a gender or lacking gender either, but I appreciate the archetypes represented in families like Father and Mother, parent, and child for the purpose of helping me to feel connected in relationships. That is not the entirety of my understanding, and my understanding seems to fluctuate depending on the level of my participation in that relationship—but this is the concept I return to most often.

The point of the 12-Step program is to find access to a power greater than yourself so you can overcome the compulsion to drink. It doesn't have to mean you abandon your own power—only that you add to it.

19

Is This a Cult or What?

Wikipedia defines a cult as "A relatively small group, which is typically led by a charismatic and self-appointed leader, who excessively controls its members, requiring unwavering devotion to a set of beliefs and practices which are considered deviant."

If you find yourself in a group like that, please understand that they do not represent AA as a whole and you should find another group.

As an organization, Alcoholics Anonymous goes to great lengths to express that there are no leaders, only trusted servants. While the founders—Dr. Bob and Bill W.—are deeply respected, they knew the organization needed to be decentralized to survive. The program has one primary purpose: to help alcoholics who are still suffering. There's nothing deviant about that! The traditions specifically prohibit outside financial contributions to avoid any deviation from that primary purpose. Also, there are no dues or fees for membership. The meetings run solely based on their ability to support themselves.

The idea that AA is a cult arises from some of the members who are either too controlling, or who don't allow any sort of questioning of the program nor its ideas or literature. However, every organization needs to be able to stand up to scrutiny to be validated and understood by those participating. New members need to be able to bring up their concerns and discuss them in a safe environment so they can assimilate the information they are receiving.

20

Yikes, Too Many Rules!

There is no denying that the program can be very rigid. But let's stop for a moment and examine where those ideas come from, and how we might apply the information to our specific needs. There are many references in *Alcoholics Anonymous* supporting the idea of total compliance. For example, let's consider the saying, "Half measures avail us nothing." It is stated repeatedly in the literature that to pick and choose which steps we want to do or to practice anything less than rigorous honesty doesn't typically lead to sustained sobriety.

Keep in mind that when the steps were written, it was with the intention to reach people who were described in the literature as "real alcoholics." Those in such deep denial and physical peril that they needed strict guidelines to prevent them from finding excuses to drink. In 1939, there were no treatment centers or rehabilitation centers as we know them today, so the 12-Step program was—for all practical purposes—the only viable option. Even though there are many other paths available today this sentiment has persisted, since many people within the fellowship feel they tried everything else and AA was the only option that worked for them.

It's also true that some members can be fiercely protective of the 12-Step program and all its suggestions and can become incredibly defensive at times. You might find compassion in knowing this tendency generally stems from their own personal experiences of having benefitted from the program, as well as having witnessed others die after relapsing . It's an incredibly painful experience to lose someone you love to addiction. I was told that if I stayed sober long enough, I'd go to a lot of funerals and that turned out to be true. A woman I went to high school with had been sober well over 10 years when she relapsed. She died of alcohol poisoning on her couch, and it was her husband and kids who found her when they got home. Her death rocked our community. We were all deeply impacted by her loss. So, is it any wonder some people are so adamant about working the program?

It might also help you to understand that this rigid way of thinking is born out of a true desire to help others. For some, the 12-Step process was truly the only way they were able to get sober after trying everything else. They mistakenly conclude that it's the only way anyone else will be able to quit, too. Give them a little grace, but don't allow anyone else's opinions to deter you from your own path or your access to this program of transformation.

Remember, the people are not the program.

The reason the program can feel so rigid is that overcoming addiction is hard! We often need firm boundaries because our urge to escape painful feelings can convince us to rationalize and justify harmful behavior that can lead us to relapse. Coming back from a relapse is an incredibly painful experience that can reinforce feelings of guilt and shame. I've seen people relapse for a multitude of reasons, often entering a vicious cycle of repeated relapses that can take years to recover from. They become self-identified as a "chronic relapser," which becomes a self-fulfilling prophecy. It adds another layer of guilt, and shame on top of an already difficult process.

21

Wait, Is This Really For Women Too?

Alcoholics Anonymous was written in 1939 by Bill W., who was also heavily influenced by The Oxford Group, which explains the religious and patriarchal influence found in the literature. At that time, it was mostly men who suffered from alcoholism, with women in the minority so it was mostly addressing men. However in the personal stories there is a chapter called "Women Suffer Too" and "The Housewife Who Drank at Home."

When I first got sober, I remember feeling particularly marginalized as a woman when I read the literature. It was "he" this, and "him" that, and all references to God were in the male pronoun. Don't even get me started on the "Chapter to the Wives" which felt particularly condescending and dismissive to women. I even went so far as to edit my copy of *Alcoholics Anonymous*, changing wording to female pronouns. However, I did not let that stop me from moving forward. I hung onto the suggestion I heard that I could take what I like and leave the rest.

Even though I found some of the language annoying at times, most of it spoke to me in profound and relatable ways. Maybe the gender didn't fit, or the circumstances were different, and the language was outdated, but the feelings expressed were similar to my own. There was real honesty in the stories: how ugly it got, the horrible things they did, the people they hurt, and the incomprehensible demoralization they felt—a feeling alcoholics understand all too well. Hearing the worst in their stories, and the hope and transformation they found by doing this work, inspired me to keep doing the steps.

Ironically, having been raised in a deeply religious household much of the language I found in the Big Book felt both familiar and comforting to me. Having spent a lot of time at church, I was trained to translate the words and lessons of the Bible and imbue them with meaning, to apply these lessons to my own life. So, reading the outdated language in the literature of Alcoholics Anonymous, then translating it to modern terminology, came quite naturally. However, this doesn't mean if you come from a different background entirely that you can't apply the same information to your own life. The way I assimilate the information is to simply translate it by asking myself, *How does this apply to me?*

Over the years, as women have gained more rights and responsibilities, the rate of alcoholism among women has increased dramatically. For years now, alcohol manufacturers have actively marketed to women through advertising campaigns that have given rise to the "Mommy wine culture" where it has become normalized for mothers to make light of drinking to cope with motherhood. You don't have to look very hard to find influencers on social media who openly joke about how they drink at their kids' sporting events, call it "Mommy juice", or display housewares with saying like "I wine because they whine."

Today the rate of alcoholism in women, as well as alcohol-related diseases, reflect the many variables that contribute to the growing number of women alcoholics.

22

Won't Sobriety Be Boring?

Before I quit drinking, it was difficult to imagine that my life without alcohol would still include fun. My idea of a good time was drinking as much as I could, smoking weed, flirting with men, having some laughs, and maybe creating a little drama for entertainment. That behavior wired my dopamine reward circuit on a chemical level, so that I *needed* that kind of intensity in order to have "a good time." Once I stopped drinking, I admit that life did feel flat—but it was temporary. My brain was in the process of healing, and I wasn't experiencing that same flood of dopamine all the time. Within a few weeks, my chemical levels returned to normal and I started feeling like my fun self again—minus the booze and drama.

I was also forced to compare my sober life to my drinking life, and you know what's really boring? Drinking so much that you pass out at 8:00 pm and miss out on an entire evening of fun. Or being so hung over on a Saturday morning, puking your guts out with the worst headache of your life, that you miss out on all the fun everyone else is having? Or how about jail? I have heard countless stories of how many otherwise successful people wind up spending a night in jail, all because they had "one drink too many."

However, there are many valid fears associated with boredom. For example, the fear of feeling left out of your current social circle is one I hear a lot. You might not want to go to events where people are drinking, but you end up not being invited because people know you're sober. In these instances, it's easy to feel rejected. A newly sober lifestyle can be confusing and frustrating, but it doesn't have to be that way if you anticipate it and implement strategies and tactics that allow you to participate safely in social events.

A good way to accomplish this is to let your friends know you'd still like to be invited, but you might have to leave early if you feel uncomfortable. Or perhaps invite your friends to activities that aren't centered on drinking. This can feel awkward at the beginning but improves with repeated exposure. After some practice, your feelings of self-consciousness will become desensitized. After all, the goal of sobriety is to help you interact in the world, not isolate you from it. When you first begin attending meetings, you'll often hear people talk about the "pink cloud" experience, which is a common phenomenon in early recovery. This is when life starts to feel good again; relationships begin to mend; and a fresh, new appreciation for life begins to develop.

There is a saying in the 12-Step community that we're not a glum lot because it's a community who LOVES to have fun. Once you find your people, there is typically no shortage of fun things to do. There are sober travel groups, all kinds of athletic outings, dinners to celebrate milestones, sober picnics, and the list goes on.

23

Rock Bottom? Not Even Close!

The good news is that you do not necessarily have to hit rock-bottom to benefit from working the 12 Steps. It's a common belief that you must be at your lowest point in every way to fully surrender to the process, but that's not true for everyone.

There is a term "high bottom" which is used by people who are high functioning, still have their material possessions, or have not had any legal issues. Even people who have not had a lot of external consequences join AA. For these people it is more about how they feel inside. A person who has a high-bottom can still feel lonely, depressed, guilty, and ashamed of their drinking. That is a valid enough reason to go.

So, does one have to hit rock-bottom to join AA? The short answer is: it depends. Some people do, and some people don't because it depends on the individual as well as the many variables of their circumstances. Pain is also relative, and what feels like rock-bottom to one person is just the beginning for another. Rock-bottom is when you decide to stop digging.

Rock-bottom is usually described as reaching a point where you are so low there is nowhere else to go but up. You're desperate for change, and there is something powerful about being in that state—

that's when the magic of surrender can take hold, where you become willing to do things you wouldn't have considered under any other circumstances.

After an especially horrible night of drinking, I was compelled to spend the next two years studying personal growth. I practically lived in the self-help section at Barnes & Noble. I was convinced there was something fundamentally wrong with me, and that having enough money or falling in love would solve all my problems. As it turned out, it was love that saved me, but it didn't show up the way I imagined. There was no man riding a white horse coming to save me. Instead, that love arrived through the women I met in Alcoholics Anonymous.

But before that, all that time I spent searching for answers, it didn't even occur to me that abstinence from drugs and alcohol would lead me to a life of meaning and purpose. I didn't want to stop drinking, or relaxing with a little bit of weed (okay, a *lot* of weed). Since I am a resourceful person and pride myself on figuring things out, I set my mind to improving my life.

I tried Tony Robbins' books like *Unleash the Power Within: Personal Coaching to Transform Your Life*; reading his work was the first time I was introduced to the concept that if I changed my belief systems, I could change my life. But that didn't work either. It wasn't until I tried things from every angle, worked myself into exhaustion, and still created so much fallout from my drinking that I finally became sick and tired of being sick and tired.

It was only after I hit rock-bottom that I was finally willing to take suggestions from a few sober people I knew, and to try 12-Step meetings. Then, and only then, was I able to level my pride, surrender, trust the process, and take action in the form of the 12 Steps. I did 90 meetings in 90 days, flooding my mind with solutions to my drinking problem and developing relationships with like-minded people dedicated to the same purpose. I was suffering from a disease of isolation, and connection was the cure. It was a connection to a power greater than myself, and that I could only find through interacting with others.

Hitting rock-bottom doesn't mean you have to lose everything or go to jail. It just means you have come to a point where you decided alcohol is taking more than it's giving. It can even mean you still have everything like the house, the family, and the job, but that you've hit an emotional bottom where you're so tired of living the way you've been living that you're willing to do the work required to stop drinking. That's where transformation begins.

24

Alcohol: My Favorite Way To Relax

If you're using alcohol as a reward at the end of a long day—ostensibly to relax—just know there are substitutes that will eventually be just as satisfying, but without the negative consequences. Practices like 10 minutes of guided meditation will allow you to relax without waking up with a horrible hangover, and a family that is furious at you. Self-soothing activities like taking a bath, practicing art therapy, gardening, spending time with pets, listening to music, playing an instrument, crocheting, or other hobbies, are just a few other ways to relax. Physical exercise such as yoga, hiking, biking, running, and weightlifting are just a few ways to relieve stress so you can relax. Another added benefit is that exercise is scientifically proven to help boost neuromodulators associated with stabilizing, and even elevating, your mood.

It may seem hard to believe now, but sex gets better over time in sobriety. It might feel a little awkward at first, but that will dissipate quickly. What most people don't consider is that alcohol acts as an anesthetic, initially relieving you of inhibitions but ultimately dulling your senses. For men, alcohol is one of the leading factors in erectile dysfunction. There are many experts on the topic of sober sex and a ton of resources available to address ways to make physical intimacy even better than before.

25

I'm Not Like "Those People"

Once I admitted that trying to get sober on my own wasn't working, my friend Mitch serendipitously invited me to a meeting and I finally agreed to go. To say I was terrified was an understatement. What if I saw someone I knew? The idea was horrifying. It didn't occur to me that they were there for the same reason. Wrestling with the idea that I was anything like "those people" felt indescribably horrible. People that, in hindsight, I knew nothing about.

I had no idea who "these people" really were, or that I was going to form unique and priceless friendships with individuals I would have a deep sense of respect and admiration for; people who were smart, funny, generous, and inspiring. Over time, I realized that on the surface our circumstances and appearances might look different, but underneath it all our feelings were incredibly similar.

I found the members unrecognizable from the stories they told about themselves and their lives when they were drinking. The literature talks about the "Dr. Jekyll and Mr. Hyde" type of alcoholic, a person who is respectable when they are sober, but turns into a literal monster when they drink—an idea I relate strongly to. I saw myself as a good person when I was sober, but I behaved wildly differently when I drank. Some mornings when I'd come to, completely hung over, I felt unrecognizable—even to myself.

A different way to view the situation is to acknowledge the amount of courage it takes to be honest with yourself, to be open-minded enough to know you don't have all the answers, and be willing enough to try something different. There is comfort in knowing we are not alone; that there are thousands of rooms all over the world filled with people on the same journey.

Harm Reduction vs. Total Abstinence

Alcoholics Anonymous states that the only requirement for membership is a *desire to stop drinking*. That's it. If you are using MAT, or medicine-assisted treatment, you can still attend 12-Step meetings. If you are practicing harm reduction, meaning you were on opiates and you are now using cannabis, you can still attend 12-Step meetings. Even if you are still drinking alcohol, you can still attend meetings.

Working the 12 Steps with a sponsor is another matter. Most sponsors will tell newcomers they need to be abstinent from alcohol and illegal drugs, but they should not tell you to stop taking prescribed medications. When it comes to medical treatment, it is recommended by AA.org that you follow your doctor's advice, not your sponsor or that of any other 12-Step member.

Another word of warning on medication: Not all medical doctors receive sufficient education about addiction. I would suggest you try to find a physician certified by the American Board of Addiction Medicine.

27

Give Up Control to "God"? Hard Pass

This obstacle often comes up around reading Step 3 where the instructions are to turn your will and your lives over to the care of God as you understand God. It might be important to make the point here that the steps are in order for a reason. To take Step 3 at face value without understanding the process behind Step 2 often leads to misunderstandings and could prevent new members from working the steps entirely.

While there is a lot of talk about God in the program, it's important to note that we define what God—or a higher power—means to us in Step 2. The definitions vary wildly and are much broader than what most people think. God is a concept that needs to make sense to us based on evidence, especially if we don't connect to the idea of faith. Evidence can come in the form of listening to the experiences of other members in the program or looking back on our own experiences.

The argument I hear most frequently is that the idea of giving up control to a higher power is choosing to be weak; that it's an avoidance of responsibility. That idea is understandably unappealing but it's also lacking context. The goal isn't to give up control over your own life to avoid personal responsibility. It's quite the opposite. As someone who suffered from alcoholism, I understood that I must take responsibility for the fact that my way of life wasn't working, and that I needed to be humble enough to ask for help. It's about having clarity of what is my responsibility and letting go of the things I do not have control over.

In the parlance of recovery, my will is what I want or how I think things should be, and it tends to be hyper-focused on how I'm going to get my needs met. My will is rooted in control and thinking I have all the information and I always know what's best for myself and others. It shows up as hyper-independence that stems from a belief that I must do everything on my own. Now I know that this comes from the fact that my emotional needs were not met as a child. Hyper-independence and controlling behaviors are survival skills that have outlived their usefulness.

Learning to ask for help has been a huge part of my recovery, and the same is true for so many others. The idea of turning my will over to a higher power means I begin to consider what the highest and greatest good for all involved is. It's about tuning into my inner compass for guidance.

In my journey to sobriety, turning my will over to the care of God has been more about how I process negative feelings like anger and frustration. In situations where I felt angry, I was often hurt because I didn't get what I wanted and I blamed others for my feelings. Turning my will over to God was about taking a step back to consider the wants and needs of those around me, not just my own. Instead of trying to force something to happen, my focus turned to allowing things to unfold.

Finding a higher power is somewhat of a paradox. Most people are taught to look outside themselves for that power, but it's my belief that it resides inside us all. It's about finding a power greater than yourself, but at the end of the day it begins with the willingness to ask for help and guidance. By working the 12 Steps, you are gaining clarity and access to a higher power that helps you to stay sober.

28

Who's Got Time for Meetings?

This can be a huge challenge for those with intense family or work obligations. But consider this: how much time would you spend on drinking? What about the days that are wasted being hung over? I have found when someone says they don't have time for something, what they really mean is that it's not a priority.

I'll share a story of a client of mine, we'll call her Judy, who often objected to meetings because of time constraints. Judy works a corporate job and is habitually under an immense amount of pressure. She'd often come home stressed out and tired, so she liked to treat herself to a glass of wine while cooking dinner. Well one glass turned into a second, then a third with dinner, then another afterwards while zoning out on Netflix. Over the course of an evening, the bottle would disappear, not to mention the second one she'd often open before going to bed.

Restful sleep was impossible, as she would regularly wake up at 3 am to go to the bathroom, full of anxiety. The next morning, she would feel hungover and tired. She would walk into the kitchen, only to discover the empty second bottle. She'd have no memory of going to bed, and her family would be angry because of the hurtful things she'd said when she was drinking. She'd promise herself she wouldn't do it again, but as she began to feel better in the afternoon and her hangover faded to a distant memory, she'd get lost in the stress from work and repeat the same cycle that night.

Here's the deal: if nothing changes, nothing changes. Activities such as going to meetings, meeting with a sponsor, and working the 12 Steps—along with physical and spiritual self-care—are often the key to breaking the cycle of drinking. And with the abundance of online meetings we have today, you can conveniently log on a few minutes beforehand, with most meetings lasting about an hour. In the beginning it is recommended to do 90 meetings in 90 days to get connected and gain some stability, if possible. If you spend another hour per week doing writing assignments, and an hour meeting with your sponsor, that's a grand total of 9 hours per week—if you went to a meeting every day.

You then have the added benefit of better sleep, consuming fewer calories, and have time to work on having better communication with your family and feel better about yourself. Another added bonus is that you'll save money, as you're not buying booze or hangover remedies.

PART 4

Reasons People Leave

To be clear, there are valid reasons why people leave the program. However, it is my hope that people don't quit before finishing the steps with a good sponsor. You can work a program without going to meetings, but I still maintain that meetings can be a vital part of maintaining recovery—for several reasons.

First, we are constantly bombarded with negative messages from a multitude of sources such as the news, social media, and magazines which can often invoke fearful thoughts. Fear-based thinking erodes a healthy mindset and can trigger old survival skills. Going to meetings is helpful in neutralizing those fears, as there is a consistent review of the solutions which can act as an antidote to drinking. We are repeatedly reminded to get out of our heads and into our hearts. We hear inspiring stories and give and receive love. We can find inspiration and courage that carries us through challenging times. We can feel supported through love and connection.

Another good reason to keep going to meetings relates to a surprising phenomenon that happens to just about everyone in the program—the Big Book seems to change after years of reading it. Things they never noticed before leap from the page, imbued with new meaning. I've had the same experience myself, reading a line I've seen many times over the years, and then one day, it just hits differently. It feels more profound, and with new significance. It feels like the book has been magically altered, but how could it be? It's obvious to any observer that what has changed is not the book, but the reader. As Heraclitus once said, "No man ever steps in the same river twice, for it's not the same river and he's not the same man."

This common occurrence speaks to how we evolve in recovery. It is actual evidence that we are changing and healing. As we begin to feel safe enough to touch on the truth, the things we previously locked away in the confines of denial, we let go of old ideas that no longer serve us. With new context, our perspective changes, and we begin to experience life differently. Words literally have new meaning, helping us to see not only ourselves—but the world around us—in fresh, positive ways.

Lastly, I would like to highlight the power of friendships. The friendships I've cultivated over the years have been one of the greatest gifts of the program. The biggest reason I continue to go to meetings after all these years is the friendships I've developed. A friend once told me that friendships are like flowers. You have to water the flowers you want to grow. By attending meetings regularly, I have been able to nurture these friendships, strengthen my support system, and be of service to others.

Through the process of writing this book, I have realized that in large part, it has been the friendships I've made in the program that keep me going back. Not discipline, but the desire to see my friends, to hug them, and to share some laughs—and even a few tears. Through these bonds, I have found relief, belonging, and a sense of purpose. That's really the essence of an alcohol-free life for me: to be present for love and laughter with the people I care for, and those who care for me.

When my mother was dying from cancer, there came a time when we had to call her friends to say goodbye. I'd dial the number, tell them what was happening, and then hand her the phone. What unfolded were the most precious exchanges I've ever had the honor to witness. One conversation in particular has stayed with me, and I think of it often. My mother was speaking to a friend she'd met at work years earlier and had seen often over countless lunches and holidays. They spoke of all the good times they'd shared and how they'd listened to one another during challenging times, offering support. At the end, when she had to say goodbye, I heard my mom say, "Thank you for being there for me, sweetie, I love you." I realized in that moment that in the end, all that matters is love. That we show up for each other, sharing seemingly ordinary moments that turn out to be priceless. Maybe Ram Dass had it right when he said, "We're all just walking each other home."

With that said, here are some of the reasons I've heard over the years why some members choose to leave the program, as well as my personal perspective.

29

When Groups Go Sour

I recently spoke to a woman who shared that she had been part of a friend group made up of a sponsor and several other members. They all attended the same 12-Step meeting, but also met outside the meeting. At some point, the group started studying other material, started a group chat, and then a bi-annual retreat. However, there were some controlling behaviors from the sponsor and the other group members. The dynamic left some people feeling bullied and alienated. She described it as "The Toxic Triangle," where there's a victim, an offender, and a rescuer, which leads to dissonance. In her case, the group no longer felt safe for her, despite many attempts to resolve the tension so she decided to leave that group. This included moving on from the broader 12-Step community as well.

I'll just point out that once that friend group deviated from the 12-Step literature, their agenda was no longer in alignment with the larger organization or keeping with the traditions. One of the traditions states that there are no leaders, only trusted servants. Also, that recovery depends on unity. Another tradition states that, "Each group has one primary purpose—to carry its message to the alcoholic who still suffers." By deviating from the 12-Steps' primary purpose and adopting "an outside issue" that group broke with the traditions of the program—ultimately shattering the unity on which the organization is founded.

If you have experienced something similar, just know there is no one group or person who represents the organization. I can totally appreciate the need to separate from unhealthy groups, or groups that become unhealthy over time. People come and go from meetings, which can change the feeling of a group, for better or for worse.

What I would offer as another perspective is that it's okay to find another group without throwing out 12-Step meetings entirely. If you find another group that feels like a better fit, even if it's online, that's a better solution than abandoning the program all together.

30

Know-It-Alls & Rigid Old-Timers

Structure provides many benefits such as clarity, support, and security. It can be especially helpful when recovering from addiction because in the beginning our emotions can be like a rollercoaster and it's tempting to rationalize and justify behavior that can lead to relapse. So, to some degree, rigidity can be a good thing.

On the other hand, I have heard stories of sponsors being so controlling they often do more harm than good—sometimes using the phrase "willingness to go to any length" to imply that if suggestions are not strictly followed, the person is not serious about recovery, when in fact, single parents with childcare responsibilities are not always able to go to a meeting every day, meet with a sponsor weekly, or take on service positions. It does not mean they aren't serious about their sobriety. Pushback from a newcomer should not instantly be treated as rebellion. The suggestion should not be that their sobriety is doomed if they don't comply. Reasonable accommodations should be made, according to the individual.

Some members treat the 12 Steps like a religion. It is not. Although the founders were Christian-based in their faith, they recognized early on that the program needed to be open to everyone, regardless of their religious beliefs. However, there are some members who believe their way is the only way because that was the truth for them; due to their fear of relapse, sometimes well-meaning members impose their beliefs on others.

31

The Downer Squad: Overdosing on Negativity

I personally don't like the term "character defects." It doesn't seem to take into account the fact that most, if not all of us, are walking around with unresolved trauma. We developed survival skills to compensate for that trauma, and never unlearned them so that we might develop healthy coping skills. In the case of significant trauma, it's important to consider professional help instead of solely relying on untrained sponsors, or other 12-Step members for support and guidance.

There tends to be such a heavy emphasis on character defects because most people enter the program to solve their problems. According to the literature, character defects are the idea that we need to fix the things that are within our control, namely our thoughts and actions. The literature suggests that we think of character defects as natural instincts that are out of balance, which seems compassionate and non-judgmental to me. It also stands to reason that when there is a problem we need to examine it to find out what is wrong, so we can eventually fix it. Seems simple, right?

But when it comes to examining our own actions, that's a bit more difficult. If I believe I do everything for a justifiable reason and my sponsor suggests I play a part in my resentments, it can often feel like a personal attack. This can be especially offensive when I feel I have been victimized in some way.

When I first started going to meetings, I often heard that alcoholics are egomaniacs with an inferiority complex—a sentiment which deeply resonated with me. However, I also couldn't help but be offended when I was told that alcoholics suffer from extreme self-centeredness, and that to recover, the ego had to be completely dismantled. I felt like my ego was the only thing keeping me alive at times. However, in the years since that first rude awakening, I've come to understand it's not the ego per se, but rather the "egomaniac" part of my nature that was often the problem in the equation. In truth, I hated who I was when I first got sober; for as long as I can remember I'd always wanted to be someone else. The steps helped me sort out all that I was—and wasn't—with self-compassion.

While it's vitally important to identify our patterns of negative behavior, it can be shame- provoking to be focused solely on them. The book urges us to acknowledge our character assets, too! I would argue that there is not nearly enough time and attention spent on identifying these beneficial qualities. We do this kind of deep examination not to bolster a false sense of pride or ego, but to strengthen self-love and self-esteem, cultivating self-respect and humility. We cannot hate ourselves to wellness. We must find a way to forgive ourselves, and allow healing to take place, in order to overcome our addictions.

32

Imperfectly Perfect: Not Abstinent from Everything

Old-timer attitudes like "We don't take nothin' no matter what!" do not take into consideration that some people are on medications prescribed by doctors. A lot of people who have recovered from addiction needed that type of rigidity and clarity in early recovery and that's okay if that worked for them. People in recovery generally tend to be extremists and this extends to how they work the program. You get a lot of strong personalities with a lot of strong opinions. Yet that's all they are, opinions.

If you read the AA literature on medication, it states that we need to proceed with caution. The literature gives examples of people who were told by members not to take their prescribed medication, often with disastrous results. However, this decision is up to you, your doctor, and perhaps a trusted advisor who knows you well. A good question to ask yourself honestly might be, *What is my motive in taking this medication?*

With more scientific research, we are learning that some substances previously thought to be harmful, especially when not taken as prescribed, are considered valid in healing therapies. Ultimately, decisions made between a member and their doctor should be respected.

33

Sponsor Hunt Struggles

Finding a sponsor who is a good fit is not always easy, and sometimes you must try several options before finding a sponsor that works for you. If you have the sneaking suspicion you aren't working with the right sponsor, you should probably get a new one. However, having a temporary sponsor is better than having none at all.

The role of a sponsor is to guild you through the steps. They often share their own experiences, listening empathetically, and will help you through challenging situations by offering honest, compassionate suggestions. It is a type of role-modeling or mentorship that has been proven to work, not only in the program but in other types of mentorships. With the advent of online meetings and groups, you can even find a sponsor who lives outside your local area.

Please keep in mind that sponsors are not therapists, and they are donating their time in the spirit of service and self-preservation. We are taught that we must "give it away to keep it." I'll always be grateful for the time my sponsors spent helping me on my journey of self-discovery and sobriety. But it wasn't until I started sponsoring others that I realized how much I personally benefited from this exchange. As a direct result of working with my sponsors, I experienced improved self-esteem, a personal connection to others, and a myriad of opportunities to review the information that had neutralized my fears and solidified my recovery.

34

The Relapse Rollercoaster

It's understandable why some who have experienced multiple relapses eventually stop going to meetings. In most 12-Step meetings there is a heavy emphasis on how much time you have. There is even a custom where if you are in your first 30 days you stand up and introduce yourself. If you relapse, this can be interpreted in a couple of ways. Some people use it to fully surrender to the program, let go of their old ideas, accept their limitations, and find a way to leverage humility to their benefit.

However, I can see how it would be just as easy to fall into a shameful spiral of defeat. Addiction is hard enough without piling on MORE shame. What I have found from my own observations is that chronic relapse could be a sign of deeper issues like unresolved trauma, or possibly a chemical imbalance. This is where professional help from a psychiatrist or board-certified addiction medical doctor is needed. Until those deeper issues are addressed, relapses are likely to continue.

In my case, the potential shame of relapse, or prosocial shame, worked like a charm as a deterrent. I didn't want to have to go through that first 30 days of announcing myself as a newcomer ever again.

In her book *Dopamine Nation*, Dr. Anna Lembke explains the inner workings of the prosocial shame cycle. She describes the cycle as starting with overconsumption, shame, radical honesty, acceptance, and finally ending with belonging and decreased consumption. I have experienced this cycle many times in my own life and in the lives of people who attend meetings.

In the beginning of my recovery, I had a relapse at 30 days. When I shared my deep shame about it at a meeting, people gave me hugs afterwards and said things to me like "We don't shoot our wounded." Or "You are not alone". Or "That happened to me too." They offered me empathy and compassion that helped to dissolve my shame of relapse.

That's not to say I wasn't offended when some of the members questioned me when they heard I relapsed. After a meeting when I picked up a chip for 30 days (again), some guy said, "Hey, shouldn't you have 60 days?" I immediately clapped back with, "I have exactly what I'm supposed to have," which ended that exchange. I also bristle when random people question someone who just relapsed with, "So, what are you going to do differently this time?" This is an important question to consider, however the question should come from a sponsor or trusted advisor, or when someone asks for that kind of feedback. I find that unsolicited advice or coaching is largely inappropriate and unproductive.

Overcoming addiction is a very complicated issue, and there is no one-size-fits-all remedy. Either people keep going and recognize that meetings help them have more sober days than they would otherwise, or they find another approach that yields the desired result.

35

I'm All Recovered Now, Thanks!

The whole point of the program is to recover, right? And we do which is the good news!

But something happens when we reach our goal: We tend to let our guard down and over time, revert back to our old ways. We've all done it in one area or another. Maybe we've reached a fitness or weight goal and then once we reach it we tend to fall back to where we started—or worse. That can be very dangerous for people who have struggled with addiction issues.

There's an old saying: "Don't let the life AA gave you take you away from your AA life." It speaks to the idea that if you stop doing what you were doing to stay sober, you'll eventually revert to your default way of thinking and living that led to addiction in the first place. I think of my addictive nature as a health issue, something akin to diabetes. Just as a diabetic needs daily medication, I need to take my medication in the form of self-care and service work, or I will revert to my old ways of thinking and behaving.

This doesn't mean you have to go to meetings forever; it means you will need to keep doing what you were doing to keep getting what you were getting. Some people will be fine with just doing the work of self-care; others will benefit from the accountability that comes from the community, easy access to service work, and a regular review of the literature.

The basic principle of maintaining sobriety is rooted in the law of cause and effect. Simply put, we take action and experience the effect. Somehow, when I consider recovery through the lens of science, it feels less personal, with no moral judgment attached. It allows me to rest my egoic defenses and receive the grace I need, to feel relief from my obsessive and anxious mind. And for that, I am truly grateful.

36

The Quest for Quality Meetings

Over the years, I have had my own struggles to find quality meetings. When I say quality, I am referring to meetings where the members practiced the principles of the program and focused on the literature. Groups that entertain outside issues like literature that is not AA-approved, politics, religion, or strong personalities have diverted from the program's primary purpose.

When I find myself in need of a good meeting, I ask people I admire where they go or I try to find an online meeting. In the area where I got sober, there are about 800 meetings per week. A lot of those were started by members seeking to create the kind of meeting *they* needed—like a same-sex meeting, a speaker meeting, a book study, or a closed meeting.

My encouragement is that if you haven't found a meeting that suits your needs, you can always start one.

37

Stuck in Reverse: Obsessing Over the Past

A common complaint I've heard from people who stop going to meetings is that they get tired of rehashing the past. Or maybe they feel like they're hearing the same things over and over again and it's no longer productive.

What I would say is that I get it. I have felt that way too. The way I got past those feelings was to recognize that I don't have to dwell in the past, but it can be helpful to look back at how far I've come. I can also recognize that I have learned things that can be useful to others. When I start feeling stress around hearing things that are repetitive, it's a signal that I might need to practice some self-care by taking a break. It could also be helpful to shift my focus from wanting to get something out of the meeting to giving back. And, as it turns out, I usually receive a bump in self-esteem when I'm in service anyway.

PART 5

Taking Action

38

12-Step Suggestions: A Cheat Sheet

These are ideas I've sprinkled throughout the guide; however, this is a concise list of suggestions you can peruse when you need a quick overview, review, or to share with newcomers. These are ideas I've heard over the years that support a positive mindset and encouragement to keep going when times get tough.

i. Look for the Similarities, Not the Differences

The human brain is equipped with a natural negativity bias designed to protect us and ensure our survival. Subconsciously, we are designed to be on the lookout for danger. This protective mechanism is triggered when we perceive a threat. When we are considering stopping drinking, for example, we are often in survival or crisis mode because alcohol has become a necessity, especially for those who are emotionally and physically dependent on it. Fear of loss or pain will trigger the negativity bias, causing us to look for reasons we should fight the idea of quitting—or flee.

For me, the suggestion to look for the similarities allowed me to set this negativity bias aside, listen to the stories with an open mind and allow myself to feel connected to others, which gave me a sense of hope. I began to see people I related to, that I connected with, who were able to stop drinking and start living free of the drama and heartache that came along with drinking and doing drugs. As I listened to the similarities in our stories, I began to think, *Yes, me too. I did that, I felt like that, that happened to me.* Then I'd hear how they took specific actions to change their situation, like doing the 12 Steps, which is largely a process of self-examination undertaken through writing exercises and sharing confidences with a trusted peer.

ii. Go to 90 Meetings in 90 Days

In the first few months of sobriety there will be a lot of ups and downs. Going to a meeting every day for the first 90 days will provide support in a few ways. First, you will have something else to do besides sitting with your intrusive thoughts. Second, you will be around other people who feel like you do and if you share, you will probably feel better. Third, you will be absorbing the information that will help you stay sober. Over a 90-day period, you will have created a lot of good habits, made some friends, and built a solid foundation upon which to build.

iii. Get a Sponsor and Work the Steps

The program is in the steps. Going to meetings is great, but this is a program of action. The point is to work the steps, and for that it's strongly recommended you get a sponsor who will share their experience, strength, and hope with you. They should take you through the steps the way their sponsor took them through the steps. AA.org has a 32-page pamphlet titled *Questions & Answers on Sponsorship* that I highly recommend.

iv. Look for a Sponsor Who Has What You Want

If you meet a member who has what you want, like long-term sobriety, you can ask them to take you through the steps. By learning how they think and doing what they have done, you have a good chance of reaching similar goals.

In *Questions & Answers on Sponsorship*, the recommendation is that men work with men and the women work with the women so they can stay focused on the steps. For people who are a part of the LGBTQ+ community, it is recommended to work with the opposite sex for the same reason.

v. Give it Away to Keep it

This idea comes from Step 12, which is about carrying the message to those who are still suffering. By sharing your experience, strength, and hope, you reinforce your own understanding of sobriety and strengthen your sense of self-esteem and your identity as a sober person.

vi. Sharing Pain Diminishes it and Sharing Joy Expands it

Sharing at meetings is an important part of the process of healing. We learn that by sharing our pain, it diminishes. Conversely, when we share our joy, it expands. By sharing our feelings, we feel more connected to others and to the program.

vii. Avoid Dating in Your First Year of Sobriety

Dating can be very distracting and take your focus away from recovery. Dating can also cause a lot of drama at meetings if things don't go well, which might make meetings feel unsafe.

Also, people tend to grow a lot in their first year of sobriety. I have heard that what you are attracted to in the beginning will repel you when you are healthier.

viii. Avoid Slippery Places and People

While you are new to recovery, it's best to try and avoid the places where you drank so you don't feel tempted. Same goes with the people you use to drink with, unless they are willing to spend time with you doing other activities.

12-Step Homework

There are many ways to "work the steps," but the following assignments are what I did to work through them, and it's the homework I assign to the women I have sponsored in the past.

For free worksheets you can print, please visit: the12stepguide-forskeptics.com

Step 1: "We admitted we were powerless over alcohol—that our lives had become unmanageable."

Read Step 1 in *The Twelve Steps and Twelve Traditions* (aka *12x12*)
Read Bill's story in *Alcoholics Anonymous* (pg. 1)
Step 1 promise in *Alcoholics Anonymous* (pg. 58, first paragraph), *Crossing the River of Denial* (pg. 328, 4th ed)

1. Write down the dictionary definitions of "powerless" and "unmanageable".
2. Write down as many situations as you can recall of where you demonstrated that you were powerless over alcohol.
3. Write down examples of when your behavior was unmanageable due to alcohol. List as many as you can think of.

Step 2: "Came to believe that a Power greater than ourselves could restore us to sanity.."

Read *Alcoholics Anonymous*:
Chapter 2: There is a Solution
Chapter 3: More About Alcoholism
Chapter 4: We Agnostics

Read Step 2 in the *12x12*.

Make a list of all the attributes and qualities you'd like your higher power to have.

How will you look for your higher power to work in your life?

For one week, write down all the ways your higher power worked in your life.

Step 3: "Made a decision to turn our will and our lives over to the care of God as we understood him."

Read *Alcoholics Anonymous*: Chapter 5: How it Works: pgs. 58-63 (to the last paragraph on page ending with "Next we launched out…") Read Step 3 in the *12x12*.

Meet with your sponsor and say the Step 3 prayer together.

Step 4: "Made a searching and fearless moral inventory of ourselves."

Read Step 4 in the *12x12*.
Read *Alcoholics Anonymous* pg. 63 (last paragraph: "Next we launched out… through pg. 71)

Step 4 is a very important step that requires a great deal of honesty and self-evaluation, which may feel scary and uncomfortable at times. It is helpful to think of this as an opportunity to let go of the unresolved, negative feelings that weigh us down; the feelings that often make us want to escape from reality and compel us to drink. It is also an opportunity to reclaim your power by gaining clarity on the part you played in each resentment.

Writing Exercise

Part 1: Resentful At, The Cause, How Affects Me, and My Part

Step 4 is easier to digest in sections. You can use the inventory worksheets available on the website, or you can use a notebook. Whichever you decide, be sure to work one column at a time. For example, if you begin with resentments, start in the first column, and write down all of the people or institutions you are resentful at, and then move on to column two which is to list all the causes of that resentment. After detailing why you are resentful at each person or institution, move on to the third column, which is to identify how you were affected, and then the fourth, which is your part in the situation.

You may need some help with the fourth column, "My Part," the column where we examine the role we've played in each situation. The Big Book says to look for, "Where had we been selfish, dishonest, self-seeking, and frightened?" and "Where were we to blame?"

There are situations where we don't play a part in what has happened to us—such as abuse; in those cases, I would encourage you to seek help from a professional trained in treating psychological trauma. However, in most cases where resentment is present, we can usually identify the part we have played in things with help from a compassionate sponsor.

Part 2: Identifying Fears

After you have your inventory completed, it's time to go back and review your underlying fears to identify the root cause. The Big Book states that self-reliance has failed us, and the solution is to trust and rely upon a higher power of your understanding.

The book suggests that we ask our higher power for these fears to be removed, and to direct our attention to what our higher power would have us be.

Part 3: Sex Conduct

Read pg. 69 in the Big Book. Ask your higher power for guidance before writing.

This is a review of our own conduct over the years past and a chance to ask ourselves the following questions: "Where had we been selfish, dishonest or inconsiderate? Whom have we hurt? Did we unjustifiably arouse jealousy, suspicion, or bitterness? Where were we at fault; what should we have done instead?"

When you are finished, it is time to write about your ideal sexual relationship.

An ideal: A conception in its absolute perfection. Free from moral defect. A goal.

What would your ideal relationship look like?
What is it that you want to grow toward?
What do you want in your future relationships?
What is important to you?

Part 4: Character Assets

After such an intense focus on wrongdoings, it's important to review assets to restore a balanced view of ourselves. The guidance in *Twelve Steps and Twelve Traditions* is to note our assets alongside our liabilities. In a notebook, or using the worksheet from the website, make a list of as many character assets as possible. Next to each asset, list examples of when you demonstrated these assets.

Step 5: "Admitted to God, to ourselves, and to another human being the exact nature of our wrongs."

Read Step 5 in the *12x12*.
Read pg. 72-75 in *Alcoholics Anonymous*.

When the writing has been completed, share it with someone you trust. This is typically your sponsor, but can also be a member of your clergy, a therapist, or trusted friend. This can be done in multiple sessions. For instance, you can complete Parts 1 & 2, then in another session, Parts 3 & 4.

When sharing the inventory, your sponsor or trusted advisor can help you to identify your character defects. Character defects are simply instincts that are out of balance. In the *12x12*, the recommendation is to use the Seven Deadly Sins as a guide: pride, greed, lust, envy, jealousy, sloth, and wrath. As you read through your inventory, you will notice a pattern emerging that will prove useful in navigating the upcoming steps.

A word of caution: the inventory should not be read to someone who could be hurt by it. For example, if your family is in your inventory you should not read it to any of them. There will be an opportunity in Step 9 to address those you had resentments toward in the form of an amends.

Suggestion: When sharing Part 1, stick to what was written. It is tempting to want to give the entire backstory for each cause of resentment, but that isn't necessary and it could extend the process by hours, if not days. What is important is to identify the root cause of each resentment, how you were affected, and what part you played in the situation.

Step 6: "Were entirely ready to have God remove all these defects of character."

Read Step 6 in the *12x12*.
Read the first paragraph on pg. 76 of *Alcoholics Anonymous*

Writing Exercise:

Identify the behavioral patterns (your actions), as a result of the character defects that were making your life unbalanced. List as many examples as you can think of. The purpose of this exercise is to help you recognize that the old behavior patterns you have relied on thus far are no longer working. It will also help you feel ready to let them go, so you can ask your higher power for help.

Step 7: "Humbly asked Him to remove our shortcomings."

Read pg. 76, second paragraph. Say the prayer that is written or say your own asking your higher power to remove your shortcomings. Read Step 7 in the *12x12*.

Writing Exercise:

In the margin of the *12x12*, note the word "humility," and how often it is used, and highlight the word each time it appears in the text. Then, on a separate piece of paper, write down "Humility – the desire to seek and do God's will," each time you come across it.

Step 8: "Made a list of all persons we had harmed, and became willing to make amends to them all."

Read Step 8 in the 12x12.
Read *Alcoholics Anonymous* pages 76, 3rd paragraph. "Now we need more action...through page 78, 1st paragraph...we will be gratified with the result."

Don't overthink this one! It's simply making a list; it shouldn't take that long. You can start the list by looking at your inventory, adding the people you were resentful of and take it from there. There is a good chance you will be able to think of people you feel guilty about hurting. Once the list is completed, you should share it with your sponsor. Then you can begin praying for the willingness to make amends to everyone on it.

Step 9: "Made direct amends to such people wherever possible, except when to do so would injure them or others

Read Step 9 in the *12x12*.
Read *Alcoholics Anonymous*, pg. 76, 3rd paragraph.

Before making amends, review the list from Step 8 with a sponsor to make sure you are making amends to the appropriate people with the right motives. Making amends is not just apologizing. You must be sure you are clear about the behavioral pattern you are taking responsibility for, how you hurt the person in question, then ask what you can do to make it right. The people you are making amends to may need time to think about things, so let them know they can get back to you, if necessary. They may also need to express their feelings, so leave room for that by asking, "Is there anything else you would like me know?"

It was recommended to me to start with the easy ones first, and work through the list from there. In my experience, if I couldn't find someone on the list I would make living amends until I could make contact.

Step 10: "Continued to take personal inventory and when we were wrong promptly admitted it."

Read Step 10 in the *12x12*.
Read *Alcoholics Anonymous* pgs. 83-85, starting with "The Promises" on the last paragraph of pg. 83.

Writing Exercise:

Keep a notebook by your bed; every night review your day and make note of all the things that went well. It's important to acknowledge character assets. Then list any resentments that came up during the day, do some reflection on your part, and note whether an amends is owed.

I have also participated in a 30-Day 10th step challenge which helped to make this self-evaluation process second nature. The challenge is to read the 10th step daily for 30 days. If you miss a day, you start over. It's not easy, but it will transform your outlook and how you move through your day.

Step 11: "Sought through prayer and meditation to improve our conscious contact with God as we understood Him, praying only for knowledge of His will for us and the power to carry that out."

Read Step 11 in the *12x12*.
Read Step 11 in *Alcoholics Anonymous*, pgs. 85 (last paragraph) through 88.

You don't have to wait until you are on Step 11 to start praying and meditating. However, when you are on this step, it's a great time to deepen your practice. You could join a meditation group or commit to 15 minutes per day to start.

The practice of prayer and meditation helps to connect you with your internal guidance—or God's Will—because it quiets the mind. It's a practice of being in the present moment where you can develop conscious contact with your higher power.

Step 12: "Having had a spiritual awakening as the result of these steps, we tried to carry this message to alcoholics, and to practice these principles in all our affairs."

Read Step 12 in the *12x12*.
Read *Alcoholics Anonymous* Ch 7 "Working with Others" pgs. 89-103.
(Sponsor's Guide)

This step is simple:

1. Take someone else through the steps
2. Volunteer for a service position

40

Alternatives to 12-Step Programs

My intention of sharing my experience in the program is to demonstrate the personal struggles I faced, and how overcoming them allowed me to reap the benefits of long-term sobriety. I've stayed sober through decades of marriage with all the ups and downs, raised two incredible young men, experienced deep grief after the deaths of friends and family—including both of my parents—and have survived many of life's typical challenges and celebrations.

However, I recognize that there are more options for recovery today than ever before, and that the 12 Steps are not the only way to achieve sobriety. For millions of people, it has been the only thing that has worked, which is why so many members are fiercely protective of the program, faults and all—especially those of us who have lost friends and loved ones to this disease.

If after you read this book you decide this program isn't for you, that's okay. I would encourage you to follow your instincts and your heart and decide what's right for you. The addiction recovery space has grown tremendously in recent years. We have come to understand that there are many modalities of healing that are equally as effective. What I would suggest is to consider another program, or to at least consider either using some, or a combination of, the other tools listed below. Some of the commonalities of all the most popular programs include self-examination, community, somatic work, spirituality, confession, making amends, service work, and a regular self-care practice.

The following is not a comprehensive list of resources and is in no particular order. This list will change as new programs become available. For the most recent resources and in-depth explanations, please visit the website at 12stepexplorationguide.com

Peer Support:

SheRecovers
A Woman's Way Through The 12 Steps
Yoga 12-Step Recovery
SMART Recovery
Celebrate Recovery
Recovery 2.0
Refuge Recovery
Recovery Dharma
Harm Reduction Works

Professional Individual Approaches:

Addiction Counseling
Psychotherapy
Hypnotherapy
Sober Coaching
Somatic Therapy
IFS - Internal Family Systems Therapy
EMDR - Eye Movement Desensitization Reprocessing Therapy
CBT – Cognitive Behavioral Therapy
DBT – Dialectical Behavioral Therapy

Additional Tools & Practices:

Meditation or Mindfulness
Nutrition-Based Healing
Fitness/Yoga
Journaling
Breathwork
Cold Water Therapy
Service Work or Volunteering

FINAL THOUGHTS

I truly hope you have found this guide to be helpful, but I realize it is not comprehensive. I know that as soon as this book is published, I will think of something else I should have included. I trust that our friends in recovery will be able to fill in the gaps for you that I might have missed. I hope you have enough encouragement to keep going on the journey of recovery.

If you are struggling with addiction, I hope you find the courage and resources you need to heal. There *is* help available. You are *not* alone.

ACKNOWLEDGEMENTS

I would like to offer my deepest gratitude to all the women who have sponsored me over the years. Maryann S., Kimmerz A., Rita R., Fran D., and Elizabeth S. Thank you for the endless hours of compassionate support.

I would also like to thank the women from The One Day At A Time Private Women's group for providing feedback on the book and their continued support.

To Marybeth O'Connor who was the first to give me direct and honest feedback.

To all the people who have participated in my recovery journey - I am so grateful for you all. I couldn't have done it without you.

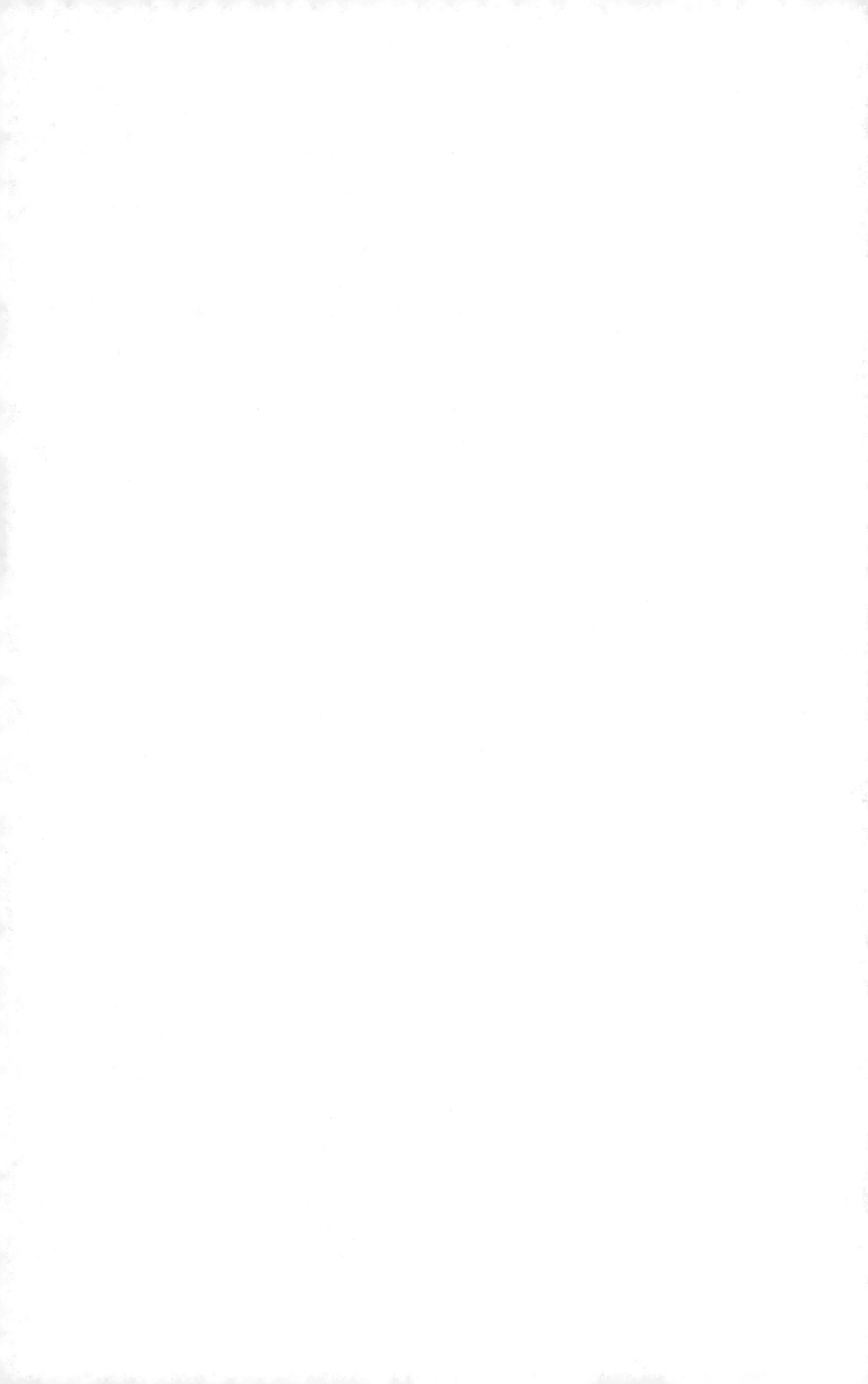